Medicine in Brief

Medicine in Brief

NAME THE DISEASE IN HAIKU, TANKA AND ART

CYNTHIA COOPER, MD

Illustrations by Pamela Chen, MD

To order additional copies of this book, contact:
Xlibris
844-714-8691
www.Xlibris.com
Orders@Xlibris.com
837712

These poems are stereotypes of diagnoses and cannot reflect the full spectrum of disease or patient experience. The explanations contain medical information but should not be a substitute for advice from a physician. They are here to serve as puzzles, mnemonics, and celebrations of the art of diagnosis in medicine.

Dedicated to my husband who always knew I could.

Tell me your story
The exam augments the plot
Together we learn

CONTENTS

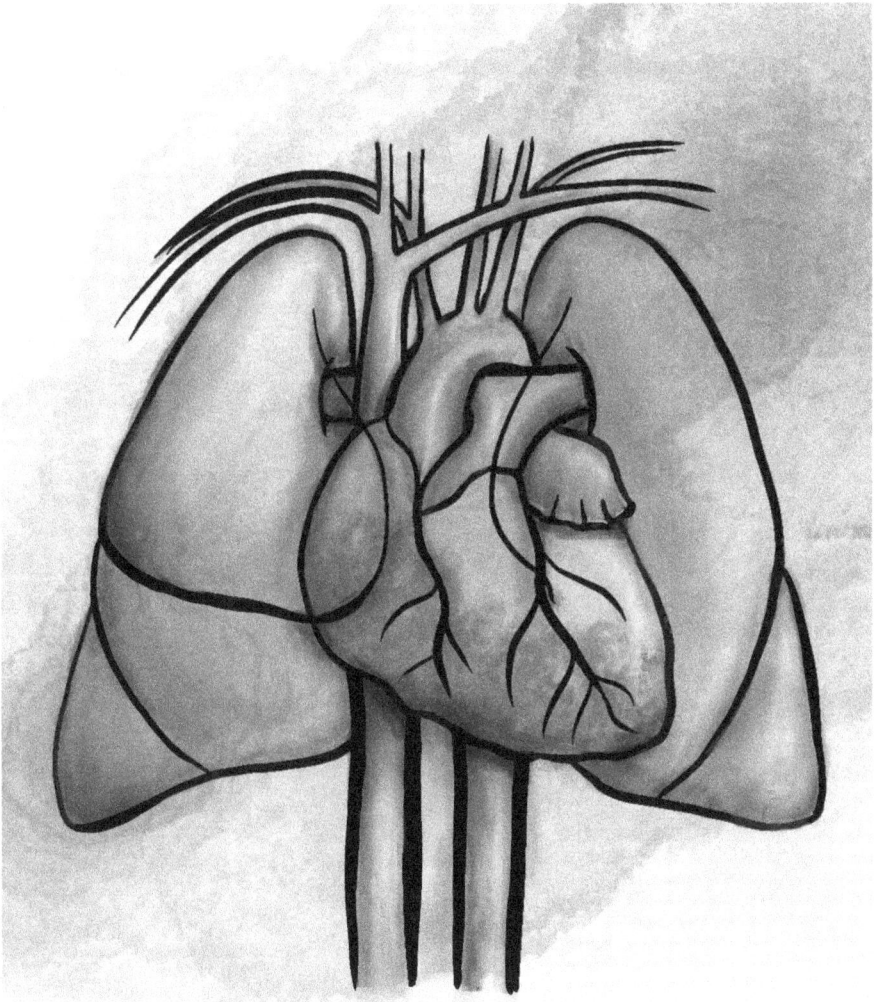

Cardiopulmonary

Cardiopulmonary
Shinhai

Transform blue to red
Exchange, filter, rhythmic stead
Ceaseless, not silent

A dull ache, my jaw
Winded with such small actions
Clenched an iron fist

Coronary Artery Disease

A mismatch between the supply of oxygen and the demand of myocardial tissues leads to signs and symptoms of cardiac ischemia. The classic history is one of deep discomfort or pressure with exertion, often radiating to the jaw or shoulder. A fixed occlusion leads to a predictable pattern of exertion and pain. A dynamic occlusion presents as crescendo symptoms that may herald an impending myocardial infarction.

Chest squeezed in a vise
Pet a cat, now pay the price
Must find a puffer
Breath extended, whistling through
Need quick act from beta-2

Asthma

This pulmonary disease is commonly diagnosed in childhood, but it can span age groups. Hallmarks are air flow restriction and reversible bronchoconstriction, often tied to an environmental or exertional trigger. Patients describe chest tightness, cough, and wheezing. Airways show inflammation. In mild cases, a short-acting inhaler with a beta-2 agonist is first line management.

Drowning while in bed
Must sit up, window, cool air
Each breath a gurgle

Congestive Heart Failure

Acute congestive heart failure with an elevated left atrial pressure often presents with shortness of breath and pulmonary edema. Orthopnea, or upright breath, is increased dyspnea while lying down. Blood volume, held in the legs by gravity when the patient is standing, returns to the circulation and overwhelms a struggling, noncompliant heart. Paroxysmal nocturnal dyspnea is a similar symptom, waking the patient from sleep with acute shortness of breath and the desire to sit or stand up.

One minute flies by
With too little breath escaped
Cachectic, pursed lips
Diaphragms flatten, suck ribs
Elbows dark from constant prop

Emphysema

Emphysema is a pulmonary disease characterized by flow limitation, notably decreased forced expiratory volume measured at one minute and end exhalation. Bleb formation, loss of surface area for gas exchange, and air trapping are notable features, leading to flattening of the diaphragm. The inward horizontal movement of the flattened diaphragm on the ribs is called the Hoover sign and highlights the loss of the diaphragm's up and down movement for inhalation and exhalation. Patients will often position themselves in a tripod position, with elbows propped on a fixed surface, so that they can use their neck muscles to lessen the work of breathing. Most cases of emphysema are associated with a history of cigarette smoking, typically with apical lung involvement. Alpha-1 antitrypsin deficiency preferentially involves the base of the lungs.

Stretched atria send
Erratic syncopation
AV node resists

Atrial fibrillation

Atrial fibrillation is the most common cardiac arrhythmia whose incidence increases with age. The sinoatrial node is overwhelmed by intra-atrial impulses, which are erratic, fast and fail to organize atrial contraction. The refractory period of the AV node serves as a point of resistance, preventing the atrial impulses from reaching the ventricle. Atrial fibrillation is a major risk factor for embolic stroke.

Genes, stress, drugs, or salt
Vessel tense, near to bursting
Dull, constant assault
Ceaseless, silent erosion
Slowly wearing out the parts

Essential Hypertension

Nearly half the world's adults have hypertension, and it is the most common reason for both office visits and use of chronic prescription meds. Hypertension is a multifaceted disease with the sympathetic nervous system, blood volume, and the renin-angiotensin-aldosterone system all playing a role. Age, obesity, family history, sodium and alcohol intake, and reduced nephron number all may influence blood pressure. Many drugs including oral contraceptives, NSAIDs, antidepressants, and corticosteroids can exacerbate existing hypertension. Heart failure, ischemic stroke, hemorrhagic stroke, and chronic kidney disease all are tied to poorly controlled blood pressure.

Every breath sharp pained
Pounding, full jugular veins
Right heart panic strain
Lungs on x-ray clear, air-filled
POCUS D sign, tension build

Acute Pulmonary Embolism

Acute pulmonary embolism is the sudden, potentially life-threatening lodging of a blood clot into the pulmonary arterial vasculature. Clots typically form in the lower extremity in the setting of stasis, endothelial damage, or hypercoagulability. The clinical picture is one of acute dyspnea, pleuritic chest pain, tachycardia, and right heart pressure overload manifesting as engorged neck veins. Chest x-ray may show normal lungs or signs of blood vessel pruning. Point-of-care ultrasound (POCUS) examination of the heart shows flattening of the intraventricular septum due to right ventricular pressure overload, the D sign.

Urine output fall
Kidneys can't do work of all
Is heart sole to blame?
Poor flow forward, high load back
Decongest, cut all some slack

Cardiorenal Syndrome

Cardiorenal syndrome is the nomenclature for complex pathophysiology by which dysfunction of one organ causes dysfunction in the other. Current taxonomy names five types of CRS: (1) acute heart failure leading to acute kidney injury, (2) chronic heart failure leading to chronic kidney disease, (3) acute kidney injury leading to acute heart failure, (4) primary chronic kidney disease contributing to cardiac disease, and (5) a systemic disorder causing both cardiac and renal dysfunction. The poem points to CRS 1 or 2. Decongestion with intravenous loop diuretics is the current recommended therapeutic intervention with evidence of improved outcomes, even at the price of worsened azotemia.

Sorry, ma'am, your husband
The heart sinks and fills with grief
The apex balloons

Takotsubo Cardiomyopathy

Named for the octopus pots of Japan, this cardiomyopathy is initiated by the massive release of catecholamines. There is impaired perfusion and ballooning dysfunction of the left ventricle, which typically spares the base—hence the comparison to the pot shape. Takotsubo cardiomyopathy can mimic a dramatic ST-elevation myocardial infarction with cardiogenic shock. Most patients, however, recover.

Sudden pain, stab, rip
Intima loses its grip
Picking off branches
Mediastinum now wide
Pressure drops one side from side

Aortic Dissection

An aortic dissection presents with sudden onset sharp, ripping chest pain, often radiating to the jaw and back. The dissection forms a false channel between the intimal layer of the aorta and the media, extending along the aorta and narrowing or obstructing arterial branches to the brain, the limbs, and other vital organs. A dissection of the ascending aorta may extend through the aortic root into the pericardium, causing acute cardiac tamponade. The classic finding on chest imaging is a widened mediastinum. Physical exam often shows a difference in blood pressure between limbs, with the pressure lower in limbs that have lost blood flow due to the dissection.

Bachelor party
Seems my heart keeps raving
Too much tequila

Holiday Heart

The spectrum of alcoholic cardiomyopathy includes acute atrial arrhythmias, most commonly atrial fibrillation. Alcohol is toxic to the heart in both the short and long term, despite some association with lowered cardiovascular disease risk. Chronic alcohol abuse is a leading cause of non-ischemic dilated cardiomyopathy.

O2 sats dip low
Lung sounds harsh like ripped Velcro
Nail tips curved, swollen
No dust, fumes, drugs, birds at home
High-res shows fine honeycomb

Idiopathic Pulmonary Fibrosis

Idiopathic pulmonary fibrosis is a diffuse scarring lung disease that presents as inexorable, progressive dyspnea. Patients feel this symptom first with exertion and then at rest. "Velcro" rales are a classic physical exam finding as are clubbed nails. Prior to making this diagnosis, other environmental triggers must be considered including dusts, smoke, drugs with pulmonary toxicity, and hypersensitivity reactions. Lungs develop honeycombing, traction bronchiectasis, and loss of air exchange through marked distortion of their normal architecture.

Building crescendo
Ache, faint, drown, death? An end so
Calcified in place

Calcific Aortic Stenosis

Aortic stenosis is a common valvular disorder with increasing incidence with age. Classic exam findings include (1) a low volume, delayed carotid pulse, a.k.a. parvus et tardus; (2) a crescendo-decrescendo murmur in the right second intercostal space; and (3) a late peaking murmur that obliterates the aortic sound. These findings are suggestive of AS but are not sensitive nor specific. Symptoms progress with worsening stenosis from dyspnea to angina, syncope, and ultimately, heart failure. Replacement, either by surgery or percutaneous intervention, relieves symptoms and dramatically reduces the risk of sudden cardiac death.

Love this new baby
My heart so full, but this pain ...
Must motherhood ache?

Spontaneous Coronary Artery Dissection (SCAD)

Spontaneous coronary artery dissection is the leading cause of myocardial infarction in and around pregnancy. Pregnancy-related SCAD represents a primary vascular catastrophe related to both the hormonal milieu of pregnancy and the stress of labor. Fibromuscular dysplasia, often previously undiagnosed, is an important comorbidity. Most SCAD patients are postmenopausal women in their late forties, early fifties.

Mask, gown, gloves, face shield
Fever, cough, isolation
Snake oil fails again

COVID-19

COVID-19 is a viral illness caused by severe acute respiratory syndrome coronavirus 2 (SARS-CoV-2) with primary pulmonary and significant extrapulmonary manifestations including thrombophilia, myocarditis, and neurologic sequelae. The virus is highly transmissible and requires both patient isolation and airborne precautions by healthcare providers. Vaccines are highly effective at protecting against hospitalization and death, but new variants of the virus may lessen acquired immunity. Many unproven and potentially dangerous homegrown prevention strategies and treatments have been marketed.

Acute discomfort
Early Vs with ugly Ts
Straight to the cath lab

Wellens' Sign

Wellens' sign is a can't-miss EKG pattern in patients complaining of potentially ischemic symptoms. Leads V2 and V3 show prominent T wave abnormalities, most commonly deep symmetric T wave inversions. The finding suggests a fragile high left anterior descending (LAD) coronary lesion, which can rapidly progress to a devastating ST-elevation myocardial infarction if either care is delayed or the patient is sent for a stress test.

Beyond smokers' cough
So young, can this be your film?
Delicate lung cysts
Is it the smoke that summons
The cells with Birbeck granules?

Pulmonary Langerhans Cell Histiocytosis

PLCH is a rare pulmonary disease primarily affecting young cigarette smokers. Patients may be asymptomatic and diagnosed by x-ray or may present with dyspnea, weight loss, and a nonproductive cough. Lung imaging shows diffuse thin- and thick-walled cysts throughout the lungs. Smoking cessation can reverse the pathology.

BP 190
23! How can this be?
Beaded arteries

Fibromuscular Dysplasia

Fibromuscular dysplasia primarily effects renal and cerebrovascular arteries but can be widespread. Renal artery stenosis in a young patient with severe hypertension is a classic clinical picture of renovascular FMD. Cerebrovascular FMD may present as migraine, tinnitus, stroke, and dissection. Affected vessels have a beaded appearance on imaging.

The atria call
Is this thing on? Ah, a beat
Wide, undulating
Lyme? Lytes? Ischemia? Age?
External pace while we think

Complete Heart Block

Complete or third-degree heart block represents a complete breakdown in communication between electrical impulses in the atria and the ventricular myocardium. Pacemaker cells in the ventricle will continue to pace, though typically at a markedly bradycardic rate. The morphology of the ventricular escape beats will be broad as the electrical impulse moves cell to cell through the myocardium. The differential for this rhythm is broad and includes ischemia, infiltrative cardiomyopathy, myocarditis (e.g., Lyme, COVID-19), hyperkalemia, and senile degeneration. Immediate management depends on the stability of the patient.

Mystery disease
Destructive granuloma
Or x-ray surprise

Sarcoidosis (Cardiopulmonary)

Sarcoidosis is a systemic disease of unclear etiology characterized by tissue infiltration with noncaseating granulomas. Hilar node involvement is the most common manifestation, followed by lung disease. Cardiac sarcoidosis can lead to conduction abnormalities and heart failure. The disease process has been described in almost every organ and tissue (see "Sarcoidosis (Endocrinology)").

Subtle slur up R
Hidden highway for currents
Cardiac "bypass"
Skipping the usual path
Loops speed with no node to brake

Wolff-Parkinson-White Syndrome (WPW)

This arrhythmia occurs when an accessory band of conductive tissue connects the atria and the ventricle outside the usual atrioventricular (AV) node conduction. This abnormal connection allows a part of the ventricle to be preexcited before the entire ventricle receives the electrical impulse through the AV node/His bundle system. This preexcitation manifests as a short PR interval with an upsloping delta wave at the start of the R wave. WPW can be symptomatic when a loop is set up, either orthodromic through the AV node or antidromic, creating a reentrant tachycardia. Atrial fibrillation conducted through the accessory band can be wide, tachycardic, disorganized, and can devolve into ventricular fibrillation.

Like young astronaut
Autonomic system shot
Gravity drags me
Ears filled scary pounding beat
Each time I stand on two feet

Postural Orthostatic Tachycardia Syndrome

POTS is a complex idiopathic syndrome with prominent postural orthostasis and tachycardia but also diverse disabling symptoms. These symptoms include heat intolerance, dyspnea, fatigue, irritable bowel, and pre-syncope. Patients are typically young, less than forty years old, with a female predominance. Like the astronaut long in space, these patients tend to have low blood volume and an intolerance to gravity.

Left prone to stasis
Clots on repeated basis
Red crushes blue flow

May-Thurner Syndrome

The left common iliac vein is compressed between the right common iliac artery and lumbar vertebrae. The result is increased tendency toward DVT in the left leg venous system. The phenomenon was first noted by Virchow but named by May and Thurner in the 1950s. Clinicians should have a heightened suspicion for May-Thurner anatomy in a young woman presenting with left leg DVT. The treatment includes thrombolysis, stent, and anticoagulation.

Not a trace in May
Upward deflect at the J
Saved from bitter cold
Treat with warmth, remove from squall
Plan migration south now, y'all

Osborn Waves

An Osborn wave is an upward deflection at the J point of an EKG in the setting of hypothermia. This EKG finding was first described through experiments with hypothermic dogs, noting that the wave become more pronounced with increasing hypothermia. The differential for this EKG finding includes coronary vasospasm, hypercalcemia, Takotsubo cardiomyopathy, and brain injury.

Before lung collapse
Could no longer swim two laps
Chest tube draining white
Films show cysts, fine walled, many
VEGF-D spares biopsy

Lymphangioleiomyomatosis (LAM)

LAM, either sporadic or associated with underlying tuberous sclerosis syndrome, can be a cause of recurrent pneumothorax and chylothorax. The majority affected are women in their child-bearing years, and symptoms are exacerbated by pregnancy. Renal angiomyolipomas and chylous ascites are additional features. Diagnosis is confirmed through elevated VEGF-D levels. mTOR inhibitors, such as sirolimus, may reduce symptoms.

Perfect sawtooth trace
Three hundred beats on its face
Rate control, ablate

Atrial Flutter

The typical electrical circuit for atrial flutter in the right atrium involves the tricuspid valve, the inferior vena cava, and the cavotricuspid isthmus. The EKG shows a negative deflection in the inferior leads with an atrial rate of ~300 beats per minute. The ventricles respond in a variable ratio. Men are affected more often than women. Treatment involves nodal blockade, ablation, and consideration of anticoagulation, as the risk of stroke with atrial flutter is less than that with atrial fibrillation but not insignificant.

Giant myocytes
Disarray, small vessel plights
Repol topsy Ts
To bring out sound, strain, hold breath
Family with sudden death

Hypertrophic Cardiomyopathy

Hypertrophic cardiomyopathy is a genetic cardiac disease manifested by hypertrophied myocytes arranged in bizarre configurations that affect the microcirculation and electricity of the heart. The EKG often shows repolarization abnormalities. Septal hypertrophy leads to dynamic outflow obstruction and can be better heard when the patient performs the Valsalva maneuver. Patients are at risk for sudden cardiac death and family members should be screened. The spectrum of treatment includes nodal blockade, mechanical or chemical myomectomy, intracardiac defibrillator placement, and heart transplant.

Problem with chloride
Secretions glom, have no glide
Bacteria thrive
Quiet or flare, harm still done
Ducts, airways, FEV1

Cystic Fibrosis

Cystic fibrosis is a common autosomal recessive disease due to CF transmembrane conductance regulator (*CFTR*) gene mutations that regulate the expression and activity of the CFTR anion channel. This channel conducts chloride and bicarbonate at the apical membrane of epithelia throughout the body, regulating water and ion transport, and maintaining epithelial surface hydration. Patients with defective CFTR channels are at risk for inspissated mucus and secretions, most morbidly in the respiratory system where chronic severe lung infections and inflammation lead to progressive loss of lung function. Complications can occur in nearly every organ, including with pancreatic insufficiency, CF-related diabetes mellitus, and intestinal obstructions.

Little flow for needs
Hard to walk, too soft to please
Pulse gone from the groin

Leriche Syndrome

Leriche syndrome is due to a vascular occlusion of the base of the aorta, often with extension to the iliac arteries. This occlusion leads to a classic triad of lower extremity claudication, erectile dysfunction, and absent femoral pulses. Patients are typically treated with bifemoral vascular bypass.

Carpal tunnel block
Myocytes petrified rock
Of prealbumin
Valve stenosis, lumbar spine
Biceps tendon rupture sign

Transthyretin (ATTR) Cardiac Amyloidosis

There are both wild-type and hereditary forms of ATTR cardiac amyloidosis that can present as a mimic of hypertrophic cardiomyopathy, with right heart failure or with low-flow/low-gradient aortic stenosis. Affected patients often have lumbar stenosis, though this is not specific to the disease. A history of bilateral carpal tunnel syndrome or biceps tendon rupture in a patient with heart failure should prompt consideration of cardiac amyloidosis.

Fleeting infiltrates
The eosinophils trail
Larval winding path

Loffler's Syndrome

Loffler's syndrome is named for Wilhelm Loffler, a Swiss physician who noted the development of pulmonary infiltrates and both pulmonary and peripheral eosinophilia due to trans-pulmonary migration of helminthic larvae. This is most observed with migration of *Ascaris* spp. The syndrome is diagnosed by the finding of larvae in the sputum. Sputum may also show Charcot-Leyden crystals derived from eosinophils.

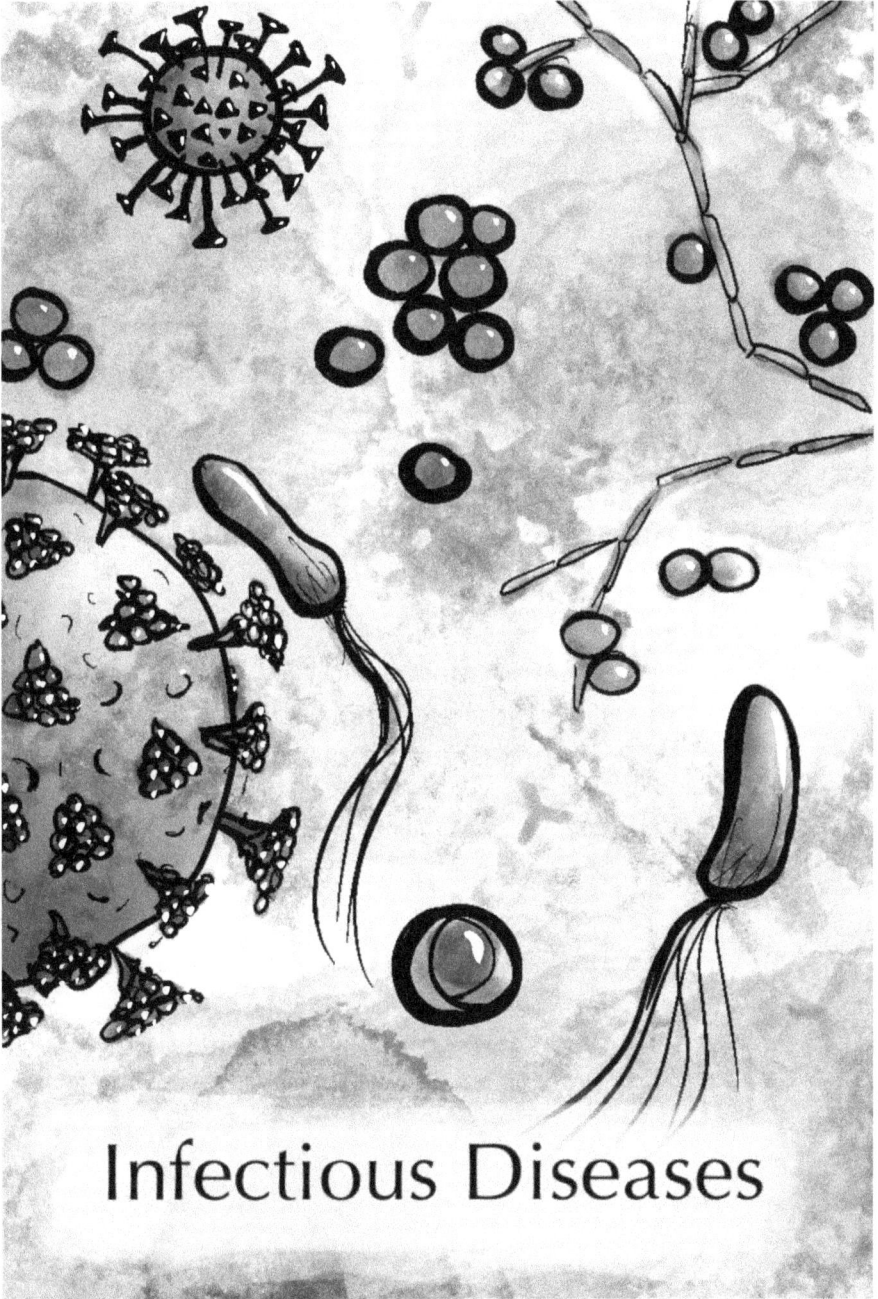

Infectious Diseases

Infectious Disease
Kansen-sho

Opportune exploit
Seeks warmth, fuel, reproduction
Then trashes the place

Sharp stab with each breath
Fever, cough, green-yellow gunk
Just lay on my couch

Community Acquired Pneumonia (CAP)

Symptoms may be subtle or sudden and dramatic depending on the infecting organism. Viruses and *Streptococcus pneumoniae* are commonly isolated, though the diversity of infecting organisms is thought to be broad. CAP's clinical presentation can range from fever, cough, dyspnea, and fatigue to overwhelming sepsis and respiratory failure.

How did you get here?
Sticky ravenous clusters
Destroy valves, joints, spines

Staphylococcus aureus Bacteremia

Staph aureus bacteremia can be associated with vascular lines and surgical procedures but often comes from an occult point of entry. The bacteria are very aggressive and sticky, often leading to devastating metastatic infections. Heart valves, joints, the epidural space, and vertebral bodies are all important potential sites of involvement. A blood culture initially returning Gram-positive cocci in clusters requires repeat blood cultures and immediate antibiotics to cover methicillin-resistant *Staph aureus* (MRSA). These antibiotics can be continued or scaled back based upon more detailed identification from the microbiology lab.

Our dog loves the woods
A faint series of circles
Such a swollen knee

Lyme Disease

Named for Lyme, Connecticut, this *Borrelia* spp. infection is spread by the Ixodes tick and often has early and late manifestations. Classic early Lyme disease is a bite-site erythema migrans rash that resembles a bull's eye. If untreated, later manifestations can develop including migratory arthralgias, large often painless knee effusions, and aseptic meningitis.

That garage was so filthy
Now so sick, eyes red, febrile
Shaking, yellow skin

Leptospirosis

Leptospirosis is a spirochete infection that is a widespread and prevalent zoonosis. Human infection is acquired through aerosols of infected animals, often mice or rodent urine, or through contaminated freshwater. Occupation is a significant risk factor for acquisition, including direct contact with animals (farmers, veterinarians, abattoir workers) and indirect contact for sewer workers, rice field workers, and miners. There is additional risk associated with water-based recreational sports. The illness has broad symptoms, classically with fever, chills, conjunctival suffusion (erythema, edema), and diffuse myalgias. Severe infection with liver and kidney injury is called Weil's disease.

Dry cough, the dwindles
The fertile right middle lung
Grows trees in bud

Mycobacterium Avium Complex

Mycobacterium avium complex (MAC) is a chronic pulmonary infection with typical dry cough, prominent extrapulmonary features of fever, and weight loss. Right middle lobe involvement is deemed Lady Windermere syndrome after the Oscar Wilde character who constantly suppressed her cough. Scoliosis and the relatively straight, narrow RML bronchus may predispose to infection at this site. Bronchiectacic changes give a tree-in-bud appearance on chest CT.

Cape trip ends poorly
Fever, low counts, Maltese cross
Spleen surfeit with blood

Babesiosis

Babesiosis is an infection of intra-erythrocyte parasites. *Babesia microti* is endemic to southeastern Massachusetts and is spread by tick vectors. Symptoms may range from asymptomatic to life-threatening depending on the degree of parasitemia and patient immune status. Common symptoms are fever and myalgias. Splenomegaly may be noted on exam. Anemia, thrombocytopenia, and abnormal LFTs are common lab findings. Thick/thin smear of peripheral blood may show intracellular organisms as single forms or the pathognomonic Maltese cross appearance of four forms.

Small kiss in Brazil
A wink, stuck food, swollen legs
Right bundle branch block

Chagas Disease

Trypanosoma cruzi infection is acquired either through congenital spread or through the feces-contaminated bite of a triatomine insect (reduviid, or kissing bug). Acute illness may present with a swollen eyelid (wink) near the bite, the Romana sign. Chronic infection can present with prominent GI dysmotility (achalasia, mega-esophagus, mega-colon) and cardiac disease (dilated cardiomyopathy with conduction disease—most commonly a right bundle branch block [RBBB]). This infection is endemic in rural areas of the southern US, Central America, and the South American cone countries.

We went spelunking
Dark, wet, cool, so many bats
Haunted by this cough

Histoplasmosis

Histoplasma capsulatum is a fungus found in soil, often with decaying bird droppings or bat guano. It is inhaled when these soils are disturbed. Infection may be asymptomatic but commonly presents as a chronic lung infection, resembling tuberculosis. Immunocompromised individuals have much higher risk of multi-organ involvement with mediastinitis, lymph node, hepatic, and ocular involvement.

Hooked up back at school
Fever, achy, gray pustule
Wrist, fingers swollen

Disseminated Gonococcal Infection

DGI is a rare systemic infection arising from a genital infection with *Neisseria gonorrhoeae*. Patients may present with painless pustules and prominent tenosynovitis of finger and wrists or with pustular arthritis. The genital infection is often asymptomatic and requires a careful history to connect a high-risk sexual encounter to the current dermatologic and musculoskeletal manifestations.

Nets were not enough
Itchy bites now fever chills
Bananas for blood

Malaria falciparum

Falciparum is one of several species of intra-erythrocyte parasites and accounts for the majority (90 percent) of severe malaria. Symptoms may range from asymptomatic to shock, seizure, coma, and severe metabolic disarray. The finding of banana or crescent-shaped gametocytes is pathognomonic for *Malaria falciparum*. Preventive measures include mosquito nets, mosquito spraying, and pharmacologic malaria prophylaxis.

Chef served rare wild boar
Scoffed when asked to cook some more
Now muscles on fire

Trichinellosis

Pigs and wild game are the primary hosts for *Trichinella spiralis*, a parasite found worldwide. Consumption of raw or undercooked meat is the principal mode of transmission to humans. Ingestion of meat containing encysted larvae leads to liberation of the larvae in the stomach. The larvae mature to form adult worms, which release new larvae that migrate to striated muscles. Symptoms arise from the intestinal phase when adult worms first burrow into intestinal mucosa, leading to abdominal pain, nausea, vomiting, and diarrhea. The muscle phase when new larvae encyst in skeletal muscle is characterized by severe muscle pain, swelling, and weakness.

Dark fluttery sight
Hit my neck, was that a bite?
Thirsty, water, scream

Rabies

Rabies is a neurotropic virus that typically enters the body through the bite of an infected animal. The virus slowly migrates centrally along peripheral nerves and quickly ascends the spinal cord to the brain. Hydrophobia is a characteristic clinical feature with the affected developing a terror of drinking water, as well as involuntary spasms with attempts to drink. Brain pathology shows classic Negri bodies, inclusion bodies in the cytoplasm of infected nerve cells.

Point pierces sole deep
Startled by noise, cannot keep
Mouth from spastic smile
Arched back, neck in painful twist
Nails dig deep the clench of fist

Tetanus

Clostridium tetani spores, found in the environment, gain entrance through penetrating wounds. The vegetative form produces a toxin that blocks inhibitory neurotransmitter release from the spinal cord and brain stem. The result is disinhibition of anterior motor horn cells and autonomic neurons with subsequent painful spasms (lock jaw, *risus sardonicus*—a.k.a. sardonic smile—opisthotonos). These spasms can be triggered by a startle and result in autonomic instability.

Life upended here
Change of climate, sick reindeer
Thaw of permafrost
Gram positive rods on smear
Warmed spores will kill more each year

Anthrax

Bacillus anthracis are gram positive rods that can lie dormant as spores. Preservation of spores can lead to disease outbreaks in regions where the disease has not been observed for decades. In 2016, there was an outbreak of anthrax on the Yamal Peninsula in Siberia, which was thought to be due to infected reindeer carcasses in the permafrost now thawed due to warming temperatures. Thousands of reindeer were killed in the outbreak as well as at least one child of the local tribe from gastrointestinal anthrax. The ability of this organism to form long-lived spores and transform into an infectious organism that can cause lethal infection make it an agent of concern for bioterrorism attacks.

"Your cat is not nice.
He's bitten each limb, some twice.
He must go." "Billy?
He's sweet, you're being silly."
Swab grows coccobacilli

Pasteurella

Pasteurella multocida (the most common *Pasteurella* pathogen in human infections) is a gram-negative coccobacillus. The bacteria are found in the mouths and on the claws of both wild and domesticated animals. The bacteria can cause severe skin and soft tissue infections but also rarely cause pneumonia, bacteremia, endocarditis, and meningitis. Peritonitis cases have been reported due to pet cats chewing on the dialysis tubing of home peritoneal dialysis patients.

Fever rash as child
Now adult, searing pains shoot
Wakened in nerve root
Burning red base with clear dome
Snaking along dermatome

Varicella-Zoster Virus

VZV transmits by the airborne route and causes a primary infection, typically in childhood, with the clinical picture of chickenpox, a self-limited febrile illness with an itchy rash capable of leaving pockmark scars. The virus remains dormant in a dorsal root ganglion until it is reactivated, by illness or immunosuppression, to travel along the spinal nerve. The result is a painful, vesicular, scarring rash along a dermatome as zoster, or shingles. Nerve pain may persist long after the rash of zoster fades.

Opportunist all
Invade, hang out, have a ball
Galactomannan
Raves where conidia fly
Fungi but not a fun guy

Aspergillosis

The fungus *Aspergillus fumigatus* can create a spectrum of disease: asymptomatic colonization after inhalation of conidia, allergic disease (allergic bronchopulmonary aspergillosis [APBA]), pulmonary fungus ball, or invasive disease. Galactomannan is found in the cell walls of aspergillus. A positive serum galactomannan antigen suggests invasive disease.

"Cool, dry air will help"
What consumes your lungs, your health?
Blood with every cough
Past plomage with paraffin
Rest lungs, smother red snappers

Tuberculosis

Mycobacterium tuberculosis is a worldwide pathogen, infectious and productive of significant morbidity with chronic cough, hemoptysis, and weight loss seen in traditional pulmonary TB. TB can also cause prominent extrapulmonary infections in the cervical lymph nodes (scrofula), GI tract, genitourinary system, and spine (Pott's disease). Before effective therapy was developed, patients with resources were sent to sanitariums in the hopes that they would benefit from the cool, dry air. Mycobacteria, on sputum smear, have been described as red snappers as they stain positive (red) on acid fast stain. Prior to the discovery of effective antimycobacterial drug regimens, TB was treated with therapeutic pneumothorax (plomage). This was accomplished through the injection of paraffin or placement of lucite balls into the pleural space.

Hidden, painless sore
Palmar rash, lost vision, more
See Starry silver
Wide gait, wrecked position tract
Pupils oblige, won't react

Syphilis

Remarkable infection caused by the spirochete *Treponema pallidum*, spread either congenitally or sexually, which is known for its protean manifestations. Classic early finding is a painless ulcer at the site or inoculation. Secondary syphilis presents as painless diffuse papules with palm and sole involvement. Finally, late findings range from neuropsychiatric disease to ocular involvement, and aortitis. Tabes dorsalis is a late consequence of neurosyphilis infection leading to the slow degeneration of dorsal root ganglia in the spinal cord, which results in a wide based gait, paresthesias, and loss of position sense. The Argyll-Robertson pupil of advanced neurosyphilis reduces in size to focus on a near object but does not constrict in response to bright light. The diagnosis of syphilis is primarily serologic, though a Warthin-Starry stain highlights these organisms on smear or biopsy.

Swimming in the Nile
Skin pierced by cercariae
Eggs lodged everywhere
Katayama sudden storm
Quiets down to pipestem form

Schistosomiasis

Schistosomiasis is a widespread, worldwide parasite found in warm tropical areas. Freshwater snails are the repository for the infection. Cercarial larvae pierce skin and grow to adult worms. These worms produce eggs that enter the hosts' system and lodge in tissues. About half of infected individuals will have an acute phase of illness called Katayama syndrome, which is a systemic hypersensitivity reaction to the circulating eggs. The syndrome is marked by fever, urticaria, angioedema, as well as dry cough, diarrhea, and headache. Chronic infection is notable for ongoing inflammation and fibrosis with the liver and the bladder the two sites most targeted by different Schistosomiasis species. Scarring and fibrosis near the liver is periportal, known as Symmers' pipestem fibrosis, and causes portal hypertension without signs and symptoms of liver dysfunction. Neurologic and ophthalmologic involvement with eggs and inflammation can be devastating.

Barefoot on warm ground
Larvae enter without sound
Become anemic
Nutrients gleaned GI tract
Amassed tiny vampire pack

Hookworm Infection

Hookworm (*Necator, Ancyclostoma*) larvae in warm, moist contaminated soil can pierce the skin, typically bare feet. The larvae travel through the body, passing through the pulmonary system, and are swallowed into the GI tract. Mature worms attach to the mucosa. The worms drain blood and prevent nutrient absorption. Infection is diagnosed by the discovery of ova in stool.

Swift start agony
Chin to chest flexes hip, knee
Fever, bright lights sting

Meningitis

The meninges may be inflamed by infectious (including viral, bacterial, mycobacterial, fungal) and noninfectious pathologies (including drug reaction). Bacterial infection is the most acutely morbid etiology. Fever, photophobia, and signs of meningeal irritation form the classic clinical picture. Brudzinski's sign is involuntary flexing of the hips and knees after the neck is flexed.

Rotten tooth festers
Dank bacteria zest for
Deadly triangles
Tongue lifted by rapid spread
Dark spaces beyond the head

Ludwig's angina

Ludwig's angina is a polymicrobial infection often originating from the molar teeth, periodontitis, or after dental implants. The infection has aggressive spread, producing a brawny cellulitis. The development of a firm bull neck and the double-tongue sign are both worrisome for potential loss of airway and spread of the infection into the neck and anterior mediastinum.

Fetid invasion
Thin sheath breached to one blue main
Foul heat cooks the vein

Lemierre's Syndrome

Lemierre's syndrome is septic thrombophlebitis of a jugular vein due to extension of an anaerobic oropharyngeal infection, classically caused by *Fusobacterium* spp. The infection breaches the carotid sheath and causes local infection and thrombosis. Patients present with fever and pain local to the vein but can also have systemic septic emboli and septic shock.

Black rot tendrils meet
Invade sinus made so sweet
Ketones bloom fungus

Mucormycosis

Mucor spp. can cause devastating rhinocerebral infections in patients with poorly controlled diabetes mellitus and diabetic ketoacidosis. The infection typically starts as sinusitis or periorbital cellulitis and has invasive blood vessel compromise, leaving necrotic eschar in its wake. Pulmonary and disseminated mucor infections are associated with hematologic malignancies, stem cell transplant, and deferoxamine.

Move from city stress
New cows, new goats, farm address
Fevers, moldy sweat
Arthritis of hips and spine
Pregnancies lost, last count nine

Brucellosis

Brucellosis is the most common zoonotic infection worldwide with the Gram-negative intracellular organism infecting cattle, pigs, sheep, and goats, but also dogs, dolphins, whales, and seals. Humans are an incidental host who become infected through the form ingestion of milk, meat, or close contact with an infected animal's tissues or fluids. Patients present with high fever and night sweats—said to have a particular moldy smell. There may be multi-organ involvement including polyarthritis, orchitis, intrauterine growth restriction and recurrent abortion, as well as endocarditis. The low number of virulent organisms required for infection and the ability to aerosolize identifies *Brucella* as a potential agent for bioterrorism.

Rheumatology

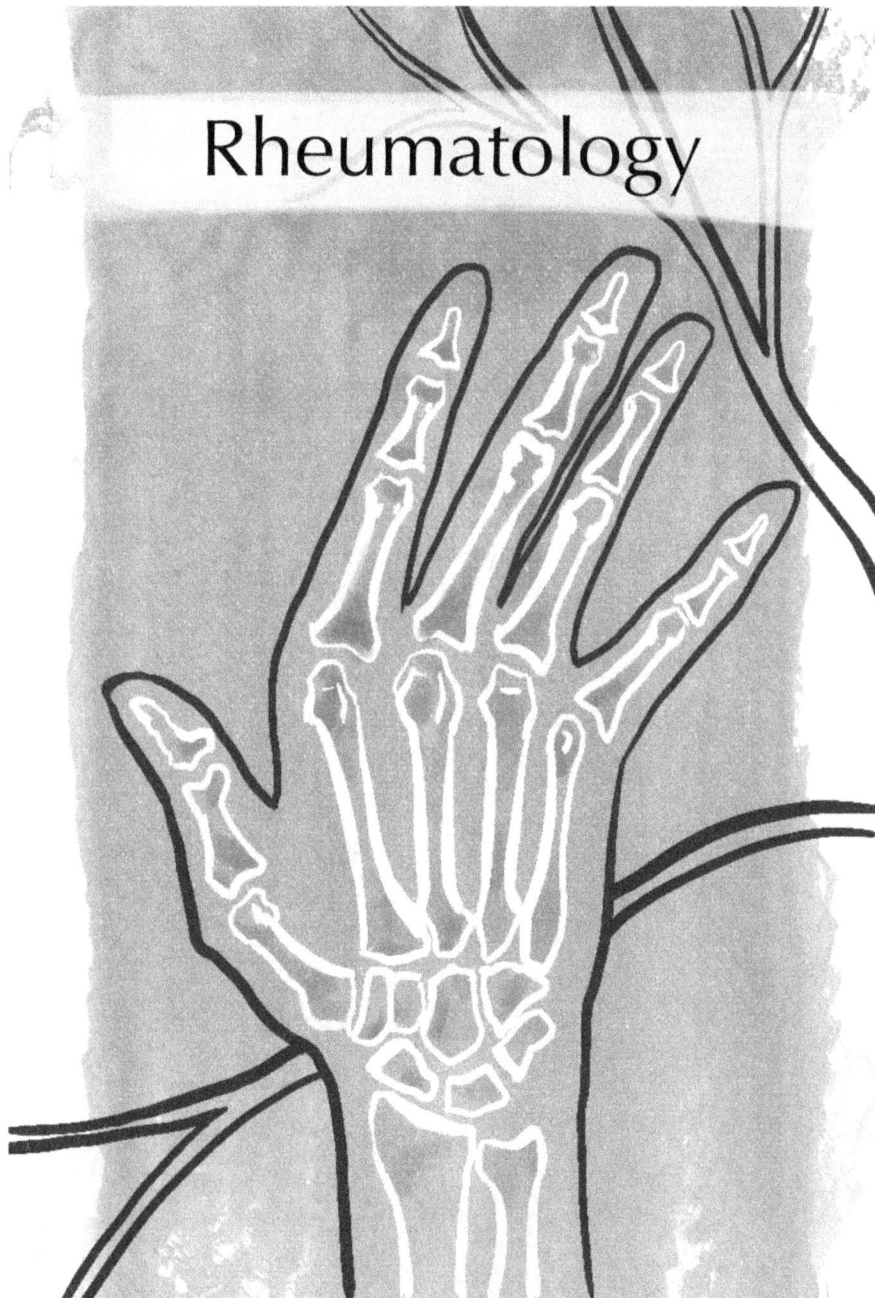

Rheumatology
Riumachigaku

Own worst enemy
A system sworn to protect
Has turned on itself

The remnants of code
Crystal-sharp needles light fires
Giant toe classic hearth

Gout

Uric acid, derived from the metabolism of purines either endogenous or ingested, deposits as crystals in joints. The first metatarsal phalangeal joint (MTP) is a classic site for gouty arthritis, a.k.a., podagra, though other joints can be affected. Gouty tophi are fascinating physical exam findings in the skin, joints, and helix of the ears.

As in an uproar
Red splatters skin, bowel, joint, more
Cramping belly pain

IgA Vasculitis (Henoch-Schonlein Purpura)

IgA vasculitis is primarily a disease of children that can affect adults. The clinical picture is palpable purpura involving the lower extremities and buttocks. Biopsy shows IgA deposition in the vessel wall and perivascular infiltrate. Purpura can involve the GI tract and abdominal pain is a prominent symptom. Both pediatric and adult patients often have arthralgias. Kidney inflammation is more common in adult patients.

Something is not right
Head, scalp, jaw ache with each bite
Flash, a quick dark shade

Giant Cell Arteritis

GCA is a large vessel vasculitis of older (more than fifty years old) patients characterized by fever, headaches, visual disturbances (amaurosis fugax), and marked elevations of inflammatory markers. Polymyalgia rheumatica is closely tied to GCA and may precede, accompany or follow a diagnosis. Classic symptoms include scalp tenderness (e.g., to a comb) and aching discomfort that develops with eating (jaw claudication).

Facial butterfly
Joints, kidneys howling to sky
Consumed complement

Systemic Lupus Erythematosus

SLE is an autoimmune disease process with wide-spread organ involvement. Symptoms can be wide-ranging, including fever, severe fatigue, skin changes (classic butterfly rash), pleuritis, arthritis/arthralgias, and renal inflammation. Involvement of almost every organ system has been described. The disease is characterized by flare and remissions. Triggers can be diverse with commonly cited triggers including sun exposure (UV light), infection, and stress. Disease activity may be tied to the menstrual cycle and pregnancy/childbirth in women. Antinuclear antibodies (ANA) are positive in virtually all patients with SLE but are not specific. C3 and C4 are typically low during active flares.

Bright smile becomes dour
Nailbed pruned, my chest so sour
Fingers blanch when cold

Systemic Sclerosis

Systemic sclerosis is a progressive disease with multi-organ involvement. Most patients are female, but men may have worse outcomes with pulmonary and renal involvement. African American patients have earlier onset and more severe disease. Common symptoms are fatigue and skin- and joint-related pain. Classic signs include skin hardening with tightening around the mouth, esophageal dysfunction with symptoms of GERD, Raynaud's phenomenon, and nailbed capillary dropout.

Hard to stand, to climb,
To grip, tight jars stay fastened
Checked CK, not much

Inclusion Body Myositis

Inclusion body myositis is an idiopathic inflammatory myositis that has a much more indolent and insidious course than others in the myositis category. IBM typically affects older individuals, usually men. Muscle enzymes are often normal or only slightly elevated in IBM. Proximal and some distal weakness is found with IBM and is more likely to be asymmetric compared with other inflammatory myopathies. Difficulty getting out of a chair, frequent falls, or difficulty with grip strength are common presenting complaints. Muscle biopsy can be diagnostic in IBM.

Day or two then gone
Hot pain bouts, dip in cauldron
Curse of family
Rigid abdominal breadth
Piercing pain with every breath

Familial Mediterranean Fever

FMF is a genetic syndrome (*MEFV* mutations) of innate immune system activation resulting in recurrent bouts of fever, serositis, and arthritis. Episodes start in childhood and last hours to days. A classic history is a child or young adult with a history of repeated presentations with an acute abdomen, resulting in negative exploratory laparotomies. AA amyloid develops over time if inflammation is not treated. Patients typically take lifelong colchicine. IL-1 antagonists have also been used to treat patients with FMF.

Liver burned by squall
Macrophage engulfing all
sIL-2R
Swollen spleen, high ferritin
What trigger set cyclone spin

Hemophagocytic Lymphohistiocytosis (HLH)

HLH is a rare syndrome more common in infants and children but can occur in adults. There is overactivation of macrophages and insufficient counterregulatory response by NK cells and cytotoxic T cells. The result is a cytokine storm with marked elevation of inflammatory markers, including ferritin and soluble IL-2 receptor. The clinical picture is fever, hepatitis, splenomegaly, multiple cytopenias, and evidence of macrophage hemophagocytosis in the bone marrow.

Hands, shoulders, knees, toes
Pop up fires in palindrome
Fine to flame to fine
Joint alone or in concert
When not hot, they do not hurt

Palindromic Rheumatism

This syndrome is often a precursor to rheumatoid arthritis or other clear rheumatologic syndromes. The palindrome is a short-lasting pattern of arthritis flare in a joint, which is normal before and after the flare. Joints may flare alone or many joints at a given time. Hydroxychloroquine may prevent progression to rheumatoid arthritis.

Despite drug eschew
Fierce hot rage at residue
Eosinophils
Skin, liver, lymphoid tissue
Battlegrounds caught in issue

Drug Reaction with Eosinophilia and Systemic Symptoms (DRESS)

DRESS is a delayed reaction (two to eight weeks) with rash, fever, hepatitis, eosinophilia, lymphadenopathy following exposure to a drug. Typical drugs are anticonvulsants, antimicrobials, and allopurinol. Visceral involvement may be more widespread, including pneumonitis, myocarditis, pericarditis, nephritis, and colitis, and is the major cause of morbidity and mortality with this syndrome. Drug withdrawal is essential. Treatment with corticosteroids is often used but evidence of effectiveness is limited.

The purple-hued shawl
Digital papules, red face
All mark my weakness

x

Dermatomyositis/Polymyositis

Proximal muscle weakness and muscle inflammation are the cardinal features of dermatomyositis (DM) and polymyositis (PM). Both are immune-mediated myopathies. DM has classic skin findings of Gottron's papules on the extensor surfaces of the fingers and knuckles, facial erythema, and poikiloderma (both hypo- and hyperpigmentation) in a shawl distribution on the upper chest and back.

Gritty eyes, tongue parched
Weak, reflexes barely arc
K and pH low

Sjogren's Syndrome with Distal Renal Tubular Acidosis

Sjogren's syndrome is an autoimmune disease primarily affecting the lacrimal and salivary glands with an inflammatory infiltrate. Sjogren's can have renal involvement affecting the interstitium. Classic Sjogren's renal disease produces a distal renal tubular acidosis that can be severe and lead to profound hypokalemia and non-gap metabolic acidosis. The hypokalemia manifests as severe muscle weakness and loss of reflexes.

Ear helix red, hot
Cellulitis? Perhaps not
Stridor each inspire

Relapsing Polychondritis

Relapsing polychondritis is an inflammatory disorder that can affect the cartilage of the ears, notably sparing the lobes that have no cartilage. The nasal cartilage and trachea are often affected, and there may also be inflammation involving the eyes, joints, myocardium, and heart valves.

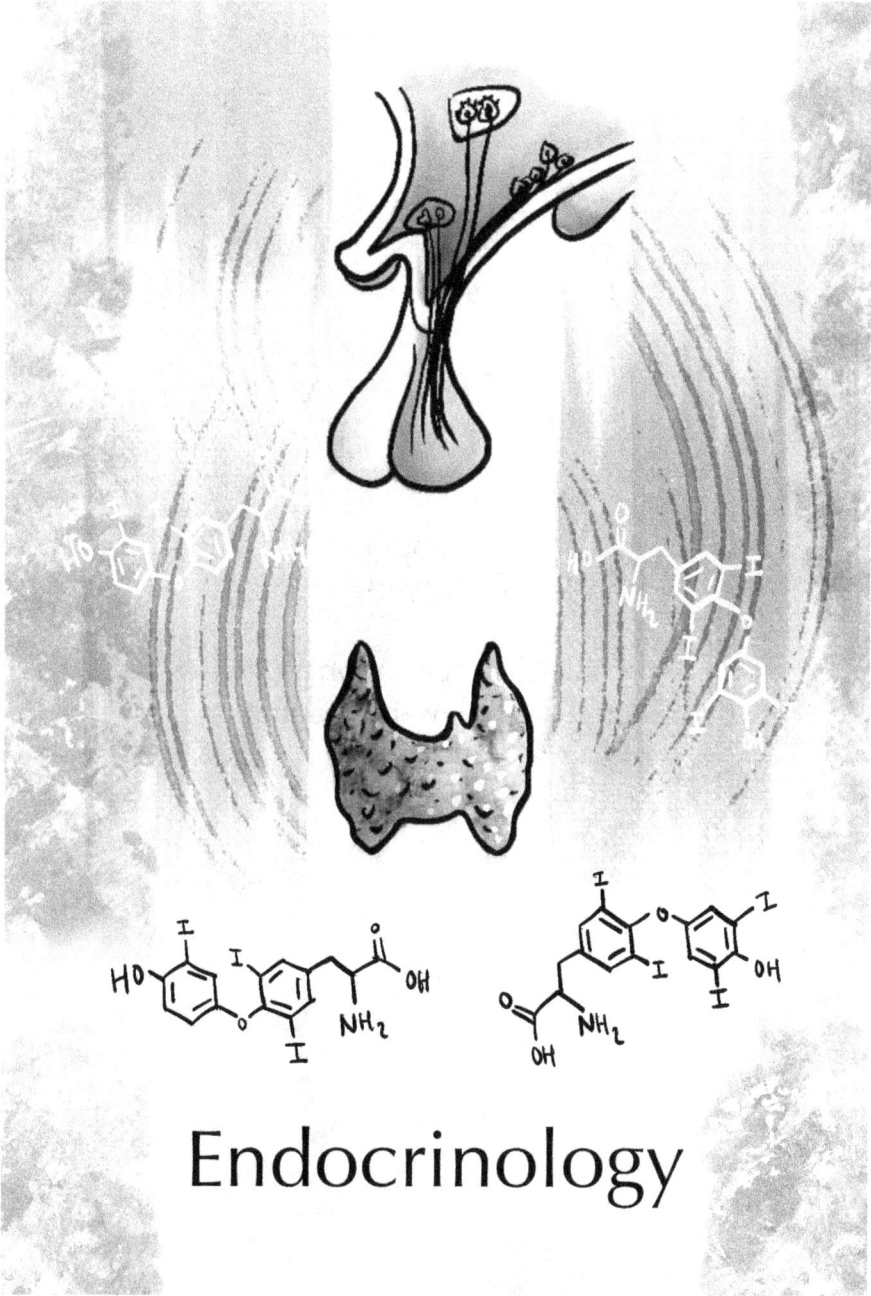

Endocrinology

Endocrinology
Naibunpitsu

Communication
Plenty, growth, want, stagnation
Vital instructions

So thirsty, starved
But losing weight, eyes a blur
The cramps are too much
Islets lost in fiery death
Crisis, chaos, fruity breath

Diabetic Ketoacidosis (DKA) in Type 1 Diabetes Mellitus

Type 1 diabetes mellitus results from the progressive autoimmune destruction of insulin-producing islet cells of the pancreas. The initial deficiency of insulin leads to hyperglycemia with hyperosmolarity, triggering thirst. There is also loss of calories through glucosuria such that, despite hyperphagia, the patient loses weight. The hyperglycemia alters the shape of the eyes' lens and can cause blurred vision. Finally, with complete loss of islets and whenever without a source of insulin, the patient develops full-blown diabetic ketoacidosis, with ketoacid production. Patients with DKA present acutely ill with prominent abdominal cramping due to acidosis, metabolic disarray with hyperkalemia and acute kidney injury. The ketoacids have a fruity smell that is notable on exam.

We may never know
Which came first, the fat or the sugar
Numb to insulin

Type 2 Diabetes Mellitus

Type 2 diabetes is characterized by hyperglycemia, insulin resistance, and relative defect in insulin secretion. It is closely tied to increasing degrees of central obesity and age, as well a strong link to family history. Low and high birthweight as well as prematurity have been associated with diabetes. Diabetes is a strong risk factor for micro- and macrovascular disease impacting the heart, brain, eyes, kidneys, and both peripheral and autonomic nervous systems.

Once a month had been
Predictable, now berserk
Ugh, my bra is wet

Hyperprolactinemia

The primary etiology for hyperprolactinemia are prolactinomas, either pituitary micro- or macroadenomas. Certain drugs (anti-dopamine, antipsychotics) and injury to the pituitary stalk, however, may also cause hyperprolactinemia. Prolactin exerts negative feedback on much of the menstrual cycle. It can also cause galactorrhea, libido loss, and infertility in both women and men.

Racing, drenched, head sore
Adrenal mass, lipid poor
Do not biopsy
Tumor made of dynamite
Erratic leaks, pop-up lights

Pheochromocytoma

Pheochromocytoma is a tumor of the adrenal medulla. Classic triad of symptoms is episodic palpitations, sweating, and headache. Tumors are lipid poor on CT (<10 Hounsfield units) and bright on metaiodobenzylguanidine (MIBG) scan. Patients may experience increased symptoms from sporadic spells of catecholamine release. Biopsy is contraindicated as it can lead to a hyperadrenergic and hypertensive crisis.

I could eat a horse
And ride one, much energy
Don't mind my stare

Hyperthyroidism

Hyperthyroidism, from Grave's disease, toxic multinodular goiter, or painless thyroiditis, produces stare as well as lid lag as prominent clinical features. This is thought to be due to sensitivity of the palpebral muscles to thyroid hormone. Patients also have increased metabolism, which leads to weight loss despite hyperphagia. Patients may also report increased energy and restlessness. Grave's disease has a distinct ophthalmopathy due to thyroid-stimulating hormone receptors on periorbital tissues. This leads to inflammation, swelling, muscle dysfunction, and proptosis.

Depressed, blue, so sad
Pounds increase, I barely eat
Purple marks my girth

Cushing's Disease

The name Cushing's disease is reserved for an adrenocorticotropic hormone (ACTH) producing pituitary adenoma (usually microadenoma). The result is excessive cortisol, which interferes with insulin-sensitivity; promotes central obesity with acral thinning; leads to skin atrophy, which results in abdominal striae; and has depressive psychiatric effects. Cushing's syndrome is a state of cortisol excess that is not from a pituitary tumor, e.g., a cortisol producing neoplasm or pharmacologic ingestion of glucocorticoids.

Everything sluggish
Cold, coarse, the GI tract lags
Reflexes slow, relax

Hypothyroidism

The most common cause of hypothyroidism in the US is autoimmune destruction through Hashimoto's thyroiditis. Iodine deficiency is the leading cause of hypothyroidism worldwide. Patients' symptoms are due to slowing of metabolic processes and accumulation of glycosaminoglycans. Typical symptoms include cold intolerance, coarse skin and nails, constipation, and weight gain. Patients may have reduced cardiac output, macroglossia, sleep apnea, menstrual irregularities, and infertility.

Were you at the beach?
Thin, chugging pickle brine shots
Tan but not a glow

Addison's Disease

Primary cortical adrenal failure, either from autoimmune adrenalitis, infection, or hemorrhage, results in complete loss of glucocorticoid and mineralocorticoid function and some sex hormones. Patient symptoms can range from fatigue, nausea/vomiting, and weight loss to profound hypotension and shock. Corticotroph cells in the pituitary produce large amounts of adrenocorticotropic hormone (ACTH) in pursuit of regaining homeostasis. ACTH is derived from proopiomelanocortin (POMC), a pro-hormone from which melanocyte stimulating hormone (MSH) is also derived. With the dramatic uptick in ACTH production, MSH production is also augmented. Addison's patients often look tan with increased pigment along their buccal mucosa and skin creases.

Something has released
The sparkling kernels of heat
Held in the colloid
Sirocco sweeps clean embers
Terrific blaze, cool spent

Painless or Silent Thyroiditis

This thyroiditis is on the spectrum with Hashimoto's thyroiditis and usually has anti-thyroid antibodies. The trigger is often unclear but results in an inflammatory reaction, releasing preformed thyroid hormone from storage in the colloid. The patient becomes transiently hyperthyroid followed by a period of hypothyroidism. Most patients recover to a euthyroid state.

Calcium in red
Since sensor not sensitive
Urine level low
Nary a complication
No need for operation

Familial Hypocalciuric Hypercalcemia

A rare cause of hypercalcemia is due to desensitizing mutations in the calcium sensing receptor (CaSR). An autosomal dominant mutation(s) to the CaSR make the parathyroid and kidney less sensitive to serum and urinary calcium levels. This insensitivity leads to a clinical picture of mild elevation in serum calcium and very low urinary calcium. The syndrome is benign, and patients have no adverse symptoms of hypercalcemia. FHH is on the differential of primary hyperparathyroidism but is distinguished by the low urine calcium level.

Sick, blinding headache
Quick, altered, hypotensive
Sella bright blood
Life sustained, something so small
Two hormones to rule them all

Pituitary Apoplexy

The pituitary governs much of the body's homeostasis through control of the adrenal and thyroid axes with ACTH and TSH are the most vital. The growth hormone, reproductive, and lactation axes are less vital for the maintenance of life. Bleeding into a pituitary adenoma can rapidly cause severe headache, visual disturbances, fever, and hypotension, mimicking encephalitis. Patients often develop hyponatremia due to ADH release in the setting of adrenal insufficiency. Apoplexy is diagnosed on MRI as bleeding into the pituitary sella. Patients develop panhypopituitarism and require lifelong hormone replacement.

Seven painful stones?
Keep missing cars on my right
Dad's ulcers were worse

Multiple Endocrine Neoplasia Type 1

MEN1 is an autosomal dominant mutation in the gene *menin*, which results in benign adenomas of the pituitary, the parathyroid glands, and the pancreas. Gastrinoma—or Zollinger-Ellison syndrome—is the most common pancreatic endocrine tumor in MEN1. The hypergastrinemia increases acid production in the stomach. Parathyroid tumors are typically multiple-gland hyperplasia and present at primary hyperparathyroidism. Pituitary tumors are less common with the syndrome but are typically macroadenoma lactotrophs, causing hyperprolactinemia. Macroadenomas may cause visual symptoms due to encroachment on the optical chiasm.

My tongue scallop-edged
A sweaty, meaty handshake
My shoes all too tight

Acromegaly/Gigantism

Acromegaly/gigantism results from a somatrophic, or growth hormone-producing, pituitary tumor. Gigantism occurs if the tumor manifests before growth plates have closed and can result in remarkable linear growth. After growth plates have closed, the persistent growth hormone leads to growth of soft tissue, jaw, hands, and feet, with patients taking on a characteristic appearance. Increased sweat and fleshy large hands are classic signs of the syndrome.

Calcium so high
Central DI, painful eye
Or just some lymph nodes

Sarcoidosis (Endocrinology)

Sarcoidosis is a mysterious systemic disease of tissue-invasive noncaseating granulomas, which can have protean manifestations (See "Sarcoidosis (Cardiopulmonary)"). Skull and hypophysis involvement can lead to central diabetes insipidus. All parts of the eye can be involved with uveitis, the most common symptom. The granulomas of sarcoidosis have 1-alpha-hydroxylase activity, which can activate 25-OH Vitamin D and lead to unregulated GI calcium absorption and hypercalcemia.

Switch from red to black
Eat too much, K black to red
A deadly sweet tooth

Licorice Ingestion

Black licorice is flavored by glycyrrhizic acid. This chemical inhibits the action of 11-beta hydroxysteroid dehydrogenase type 2, which degrades cortisol to cortisone. When not degraded by 11-HSD type 2, cortisol provides an overwhelming positive signal to the aldosterone receptor. The subsequent clinical picture includes hypertension, hypokalemia, and metabolic alkalosis. Hypokalemia may lead to cardiac arrhythmias.

Every synapse slow
GI tract refuse to flow
Bones melt like glaciers
Urine crystals coalesce
Sharpness of mind dull at best

Hypercalcemia

The most common causes of hypercalcemia are primary hyperparathyroidism and hypercalcemia of malignancy. The destruction of bone (melting like glaciers) in the tanka would be consistent with either etiology. Primary hyperparathyroidism is more commonly diagnosed in ambulatory patients while malignancy-associated hypercalcemia is more likely to be severe and associated with hospitalization. Hypercalcemia slows nerve and muscle action potential conduction and leads to hypercalciuria, which can result in calcium nephrolithiasis.

Gastroenterology & Hepatology

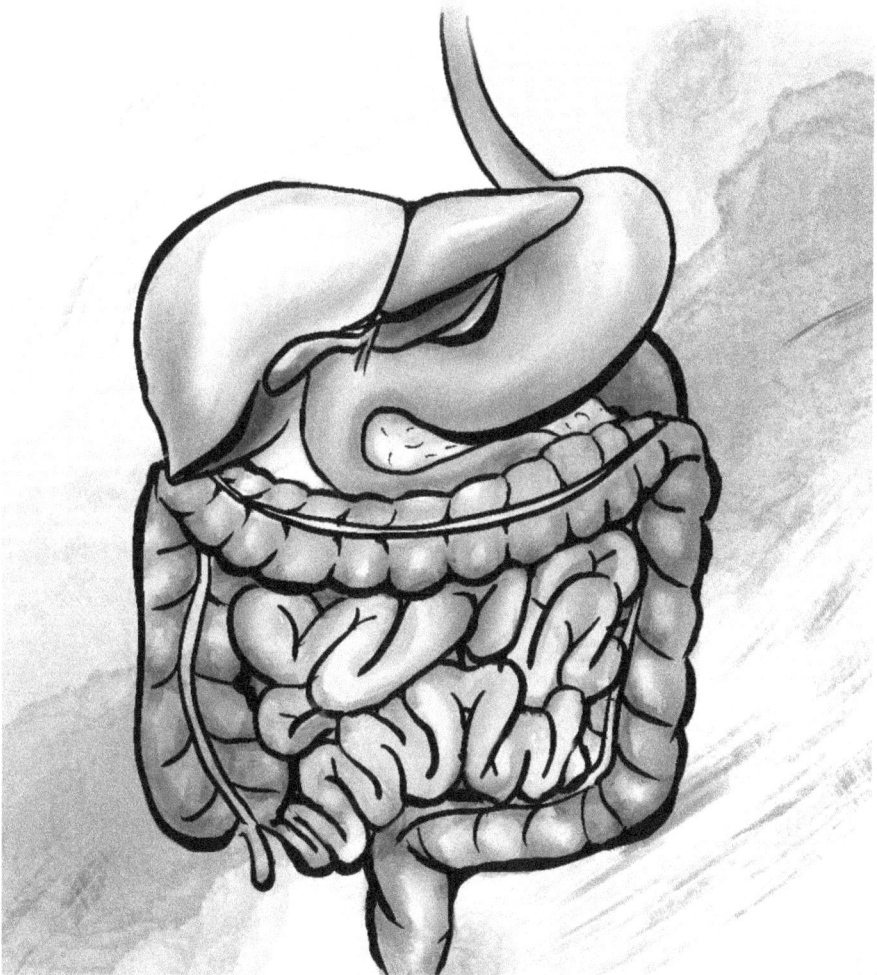

Gastroenterology/Hepatology
Ichobyogaku/Kanzo-gaku

Hollow pipe adorned
Design turns food into fuel
And discards the rest

Hung over, retching
A bright-red splash alarms all
Hard to find with scope

Mallory-Weiss Tears

With repeated retching or vomiting, linear tears can form at the junction between the esophagus and the stomach. Retching of any etiology may cause these lesions, but they have been associated with heavy alcohol use. The lacerations can bleed, producing worrisome hematemesis that is usually self-limited. Most tears will stop bleeding spontaneously and may be difficult to identify at the time of endoscopy.

Gallstone or stiff drinks
Provoked spill, caustic enzymes
Cook fragile tissues

Pancreatitis

Gallstone obstruction and chronic heavy alcohol use are the usual etiologies for pancreatic inflammation leading to inappropriate activation of digestive enzymes with destruction of pancreatic and surrounding tissues. Other important etiologies include hypertriglyceridemia, autoimmune pancreatitis secondary to IgG4 disease, and medication induced. Scorpion bite from *Tityus trinitatis*, a scorpion native to Trinidad, is a very rare cause of pancreatitis.

Spiders dot the chest
Rosy palms, ropy vessels
Fluids coalesce

Cirrhosis

Cirrhosis is characterized by advanced liver fibrosis and the formation of regenerative nodules. Cirrhosis results in both the loss of hepatic metabolic function and the development of anatomic barriers to splanchnic blood flow. Spider angioma and palmar erythema are attributed to hyperestrogenism, though nitric oxide may play a role in palmar erythema. Varices and ascites are signs of portal hypertension. In 2017, viral etiologies of cirrhosis caused the most deaths. Nonalcoholic fatty liver disease (NAFLD) was the highest prevalent etiology. Regardless of the cause, end-stage liver disease shares features of portal hypertension with ascites and risk for GI bleed, hyperestrogenism, muscle wasting, hepatic encephalopathy, and predisposition to infection.

Irregular lump
Worrying away, engulfed
Swept into the stream
Upside down and wrong side right
Fleshy target marks the site

Intestinal Intussusception

Intussusception in adults is uncommon. A mucosal irregularity, either benign like a Meckel's diverticulum or, more commonly, a malignancy, is pulled into the bowel by peristalsis. The patient presents with severe crampy pain. A target sign on CT can identify the site of obstruction where a surgeon needs to intervene before the involved bowel loses its blood supply.

Silent ooze depletes
Argon plasma lightly heats
Ripe watermelon

Gastric Antral Vascular Ectasia (GAVE)

GAVE is also called watermelon stomach for the linear vascular stripes emanating from the pylorus. Patients may present with acute upper GI bleed but more often present with occult bleeding and marked iron-deficiency anemia. GAVE may occur alone but has been associated with cirrhosis and systemic sclerosis. Argon plasma coagulation can obliterate the ectasias and reduce the amount of bleeding.

Words warp in my mouth
Red palms quiver; alk phos down
Turn my blue eyes brown?

Wilson Disease

Wilson disease is a disease of copper overload with broad symptoms, including neuropsychiatric (dysarthria), ophthalmologic (brown Kayser Fleischer rings), hepatic (acute liver failure with low alkaline phosphatase), hematologic (Coombs-negative hemolytic anemia), and renal (Fanconi's syndrome). An alkaline phosphatase (IU/L) to total bilirubin (mg/dl) ratio <4 is sensitive and specific for diagnosing fulminant Wilson disease. Most patients present between the ages of five and thirty-five years old.

Gone desire to nosh
Now, the chest filled, slowly slosh
No more restaurants
Into stomach, food just ekes
Barium test shows bird's beak

Achalasia

Achalasia is the slow loss of the lower esophageal sphincter's ability to relax from its tonic constriction. This leads to progressive dysphagia to solids and liquids. Food collects in a dilated esophagus and either slowly passes through the sphincter or is regurgitated by the patient. Patients often note difficulty belching and weight loss. Imaging with barium swallow shows a typical bird's-beak narrowing at the gastroesophageal junction. Achalasia is idiopathic, though there have been associations made to latent viral infections such as HSV and VZV. Chagas's disease can present with similar esophageal findings as can a malignancy, e.g., pseudoachalasia.

Bile ducts pruned to stumps
Elbows, eyes with lipid lumps
Everything itches
Alk phos rise at rapid pace
AMA near every case

Primary Biliary Cholangitis

Pruritus and extreme fatigue are the two most prominent symptoms of primary biliary cholangitis, the most common autoimmune liver disease in the US. Bile ducts are attacked by an autoimmune inflammatory infiltrate, which prunes and destroys the ducts. Progressive intrahepatic duct destruction leads to cholestasis. Patients may have marked elevations in their lipids, leading to findings of xanthomas and xanthelasma. Interestingly, the elevated lipids do not seem to increase cardiovascular risk in these patients. The anti-mitochondrial antibody is its key serology with nearly every PBC (95 percent) patient having a positive test. An isolated elevated alkaline phosphatase is the laboratory signature of early disease.

Contiguous slough
Blood, discomfort, tenesmus
When I stopped smoking

Ulcerative Colitis

UC is an autoimmune inflammatory disease limited to the colonic mucosa. It commonly begins with disease in the rectum and ascends proximally without breaks. Patients present with diarrhea, which is often bloody, accompanied by crampy abdominal pain, incontinence, and tenesmus. Tenesmus is the urgent sensation of needing to defecate. UC has been associated with extraintestinal manifestations, including arthritis, uveitis, erythema nodosum, and pyoderma gangrenosum. Cigarette smoking may be protective as UC as some patients have onset after quitting and symptoms can improve with resumption of smoking.

Slow invasion fat
Waistline, liver habitat
Sets up fibrosis
CT dark, ultrasound bright
Not so healthy appetite

Nonalcoholic Steatohepatitis

One quarter of the world's population is estimated to be affected by nonalcoholic fatty liver disease. One quarter of NAFLD is thought to have nonalcoholic steatohepatitis with evidence of inflammation and progressive fibrosis. NASH is associated with obesity, metabolic syndrome, and is a leading indication for liver transplant in women. Hepatocellular carcinoma is associated with both NAFLD and NASH. The typical finding of NAFLD and NASH on CT scan is a liver that is hypoattenuated (dark) in comparison to the fat-free spleen. On ultrasound, the fatty liver has an echogenicity that exceeds that of the spleen and adjacent renal cortex.

Flat cells elongate
Reprogram, a change of fate
Acid splash leaves mark
Lax, stretched, scarred, or out of place
Red tongues at change of surface

Barrett's Esophagus

Squamous epithelium at the gastroesophageal junction undergoes metaplasia to become columnar intestinal epithelia under the stress of repeated exposure to stomach acid. Patients with gastroesophageal reflux disease (GERD) are at risk for developing this precancerous change and should be screened for the development of adenocarcinoma. Changes to the lower esophageal sphincter including laxity, scarring from infection, or inflammation or displacement as with a hiatal hernia all increase the risk of acid reflux. Barrett's esophagus appears as tongues of red intestinal epithelium extending from the gastroesophageal junction into the pink squamous epithelium of the esophagus.

Neuron nemesis
Ammoniagenesis
Rough liver, low K
Starts subtle, day night reverse
Incessant flap, coma, hearse

Hepatic Encephalopathy

This morbid encephalopathic process is progressive with decline in liver function. Patients initially present with mild cognitive defects and sleep disturbance. With progression, they may show the flapping tremor of asterixis, confusion, and, ultimately, coma. Ammonia is one of several gut-derived neurotoxins that circulate in the absence of liver clearance. Hypokalemia can be a precipitant as it promotes renal tubular ammoniagenesis.

Villi are blunted
Vague bloat, energy shunted
No iron for pep

Celiac Disease

Celiac disease is an autoimmune gastrointestinal disease due to the production of anti-transglutaminase A and anti-gliadin antibodies. Patients develop an intolerance to gluten, common in many grains. The resulting inflammation blunts small intestine villi resulting in loss of absorptive capacity and vitamin deficiencies, as well as iron-deficiency anemia. Classic symptoms include diarrhea with signs of malabsorption. Some patients have primarily extraintestinal symptoms including dermatitis herpetiformis and arthritis. Without removal of gluten from the diet, the inflammation may progress to the development of an enteropathy-associated T-cell lymphoma (EATL).

Caught by Spider-Man
Smooth beefy tongue's painful span
Weak blood, spoons for nails
Mouth corners crack villain's grin
Web to catch more iron in?

Plummer-Vinson Syndrome (Paterson-Brown Kelly)

Plummer-Vinson syndrome, or Paterson-Brown Kelly in the UK, is a triad of an esophageal web(s), dysphagia, and iron-deficiency anemia. Iron deficiency plays an important role in the pathophysiology though the full etiology of the syndrome remains unknown. Glossitis, koilonychia (spoon nails), and angular stomatitis are additional clinical features. There is an increased risk of development of squamous cell carcinoma of the pharynx and proximal esophagus.

Small colon annex
Little bulk, the need to flex
Pops open these rooms
Sudden bleeds raise the profile
Blocked egress breeds flora vile

Colonic Diverticulosis/Diverticulitis

Diverticula are small outpouchings of the colon formed by straining and a low-bulk diet. Most diverticuli are in the sigmoid and descending colon. Right-sided disease may be familial. Diverticuli are often clinically silent but may become apparent when a bleed causes hematochezia. Obstruction of diverticuli can lead to abdominal pain, festering infection, inflammation, and may result in perforation with abscess. Prior recommendations to avoid seeds and nuts have not been demonstrated to reduce the incidence of diverticulitis.

Ate with too much glee
Cocktails, peppermints, coffee
Water brash since then

Gastroesophageal Reflux Disease (GERD)

A lax lower esophageal sphincter (LES) can allow low-pH gastric fluid into the esophagus, causing burning discomfort and reflex hypersalivation, or water brash. Large meals, recumbency, coffee, mint, chocolate, and calcium-channel blockers all reduce the tone of the LES. Displacement of the LES into the chest, as with a hiatal hernia, also reduces its tone. Chronic GERD can lead to laryngitis, chronic cough, Barrett's esophagus, and esophageal adenocarcinoma.

Liver warp and weft
Opens shunts right to left
Breathless at incline

Hepatopulmonary Syndrome

Hepatopulmonary syndrome is a rare complication of cirrhosis. Pulmonary vascular shunts are created and dilated in the setting of cirrhosis with portal hypertension. These shunts allow deoxygenated blood to bypass the pulmonary capillary and alveolar system, lowering the oxygen content of arterial blood. Platypnea, or dyspnea while sitting upright, and orthodeoxia, or a drop in oxygen saturation with sitting/standing up, are a classic symptom and exam finding, respectively. Patients typically have prominent spider nevi and clubbing. HPS can be diagnosed by transthoracic echocardiogram with agitated saline showing delayed bubbles in the left atrium.

GI tract attack
Running, cramping daily fact
Ulcers through and through
Disease presents stern to stem
Pyoderm gangrenosum

Crohn's Disease

Crohn's disease in an autoimmune disease affecting the length of the GI tract. The main lesion is a transmural ulcer, which extends through all layers of the intestine and can form abscesses and fistulae to surrounding structures such as the skin, vagina, and bladder. The main symptoms are crampy abdominal pain and diarrhea. Oral involvement involves aphthous ulcers and mouth pain. Extraintestinal manifestations may include arthritis, uveitis, erythema nodosum, and pyoderma gangrenosum.

Night out hope to chill
Have nose spray, allergy pill
Chewing carefully
Tiny bites, water to follow
Food stuck when try to swallow

Eosinophilic Esophagitis

Eosinophilic esophagitis is a syndrome of esophageal dysfunction with prominent tissue eosinophilia, diagnosed after other causes of esophageal eosinophilia have been ruled out. Most patients have an underlying history of atopy, including food allergies, environmental allergies, asthma, and atopic dermatitis. Dysphagia, food impactions, and chest pain are prominent clinical features. Spontaneous esophageal perforation, perforation, and tears during endoscopy have all been reported. Endoscopy may show stacked circular rings (a feline esophagus), strictures, linear furrows, and white papules, consistent with eosinophilic abscesses.

Subtle yellow tinge
Enzyme slowed, enough to tell
Just a bit unwell

Gilbert's Syndrome

Gilbert's syndrome is marked by slowed conjugation of indirect to direct bilirubin due to impairment of glucuronidation enzymatic action. The syndrome was first described by Augustus Nicolas Gilbert in 1901. Patients are typically asymptomatic but may develop mild jaundice with indirect bilirubin at times of fasting, dehydration, or illness. The differential diagnosis for indirect hyperbilirubinemia includes hemolysis.

Bronze the skin, liver
Myocytes lose their quiver
Poison to beta cells

Hemochromatosis

Iron overload or hemochromatosis may either be secondary (including repeated blood transfusions and alcohol abuse) or hereditary. Hereditary hemochromatosis is due to mutations in the human homeostatic iron regulator protein, encoded by the *HFE* gene, which regulates iron absorption. Excess iron accumulates in the skin, leading to bronze discoloration, and in many organs, including the liver, pituitary, gonads, and heart. Pancreatic involvement leads to beta cell destruction and the development of so-called bronze diabetes. Patients often present with cirrhosis, polyarthropathy, heart failure, and hypogonadism.

Nephrology

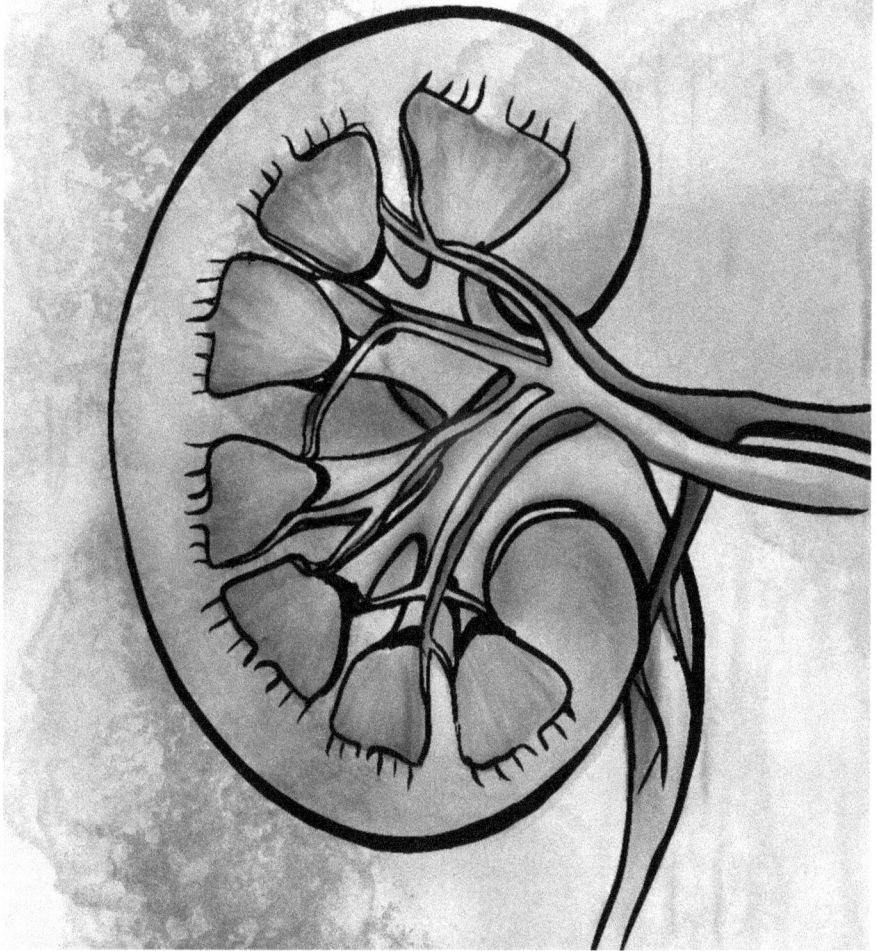

Nephrology
Jinzo-gaku

Fantastic filters
Reclaim, maintain blood's balance
Awash in volume

The liver's distress
Puts the beans under duress
How can we reverse?
Constrict gut, support system
Juice kidneys with albumin

Hepatorenal Syndrome Type 1

Hepatorenal syndrome is a feared complication of severe liver disease with portal hypertension. Damage from the sheer forces of portal hypertension leads to nitric oxide release with splanchnic pooling, systemic vasodilation, and a drop in cardiac output. All these factors lead the kidneys to perceive an extreme prerenal state. The clinical picture is one of oliguric/anuric acute kidney injury with bland sediment and sodium avidity, which does not respond to albumin loading alone. The added combination of midodrine, to support the systemic circulation, and octreotide, to constrict splanchnic vessels, might help. HRS is one of many potential causes for AKI in a patient with severe liver disease, and other causes must be ruled out prior to its diagnosis. HRS type 2 is a subacute form of renal insufficiency marked by repeated azotemia with attempts to diurese the cirrhotic patient. HRS 2 patients are deemed to have diuretic-resistant ascites.

Such weighty ballast
Cysts of no function, no help
Crowding out the good

Autosomal Dominant Polycystic Kidney Disease

This genetic illness leads to progressive nonfunctioning cyst formation and distortion of the normal architecture of the kidneys. The kidneys often grow to fill much of the abdominal cavity as the patient reaches their forties, with most of the normal working nephrons crowded into dysfunction. Cysts may hemorrhage or become infected. Ultimately, patients may progress to end-stage kidney disease and require single or double native nephrectomy to gain space for their transplant. Tolvaptan has been approved to slow progression of cyst formation.

Throb, grimace, tight chin
Dense AKI, onion skin
High dose captopril

Scleroderma Renal Crisis

SRC is an early complication of systemic sclerosis noted for the development of a thrombotic microangiopathy with severe hypertension, acute kidney injury (AKI), and onion skin changes to blood vessels on renal biopsy. Steroids may be an inciting factor. Angiotensin converting enzyme inhibitors (ACEi) are the drug of choice for SRC and should be continued indefinitely, even if the patient requires dialysis or recovers from the AKI.

Volume down so slight
Gradient in all its might
Drug works in cortex
Drink more water in than pee
Slow slide osmolality

Hydrochlorothiazide-Induced Hyponatremia

Thiazide diuretics cause hyponatremia more often than loop diuretics. The etiology for the hyponatremia is multifactorial with thiazides (1) inhibiting water clearance by blocking the sodium/chloride transporter in the distal tubule and (2) inducing a degree of volume depletion. This volume depletion, in turn, stimulates both the renin-angiotensin-aldosterone system (RAAS), increasing proximal reabsorption, and anti-diuretic hormone (ADH), triggering water reabsorption into a maximally concentrated medulla. Ultimately, this leads to impaired water excretion and the development of hyponatremia. Loop diuretics, by contrast, disrupt the medullary concentration gradient and prevent the excretion of concentrated urine. Patients with hydrochlorothiazide-induced hyponatremia tend to be elderly, with women more often affected than men.

Slow dents on my legs
Sudden sharp ache to my flank
Urine so frothy

Membranous Nephropathy

Membranous nephropathy (MN) is the most common cause of nephrotic syndrome in adults. Most cases are idiopathic with a minority caused by hepatitis B infection, systemic lupus erythematosus or malignancy. Onset of nephrotic range proteinuria and edema is usually insidious, over months. MN is highly associated with thrombophilia, presumably from loss of anti-thrombin III as a protein in the urine, and venous thrombosis, classically of the renal vein. Most idiopathic MN has serology positive for anti-phospholipase A2 (anti-PLA2) and can be diagnosed without biopsy.

What hell stomachs wreak
pH high, shaky, so weak
No urine chloride

Metabolic Alkalosis (Gastric Losses)

Early in vomiting (or with losses from a nasogastric tube), the lost gastric hydrochloric acid (HCl) leaves behind excess bicarbonate which is filtered and excreted with sodium and potassium. With continued losses, the renin angiotensin aldosterone system (RAAS) is activated, and late urine of vomiting is electrolyte-poor with low pH, low sodium, and low chloride. With RAAS on, the kidneys have a higher threshold for reabsorbing bicarbonate and the metabolic alkalosis is sustained. The low urine chloride identifies the metabolic alkalosis as one which will correct with the administration of IV sodium chloride.

What antigen made
White cells surround and invade
Innocent tubules?

Acute Interstitial Nephritis

AIN produces kidney injury through inflammatory white cells surrounding and invading the kidney's interstitium and tubules. Most cases are due to drug reactions with antibiotics, NSAIDs and PPIs the leading offenders. The remaining cases are nearly evenly split between infections, idiopathic, and other systemic illness. Many patients have few symptoms, though fever, rash, arthralgias, and peripheral eosinophilia are important clues in those who present with symptoms. Urinary eosinophils are neither sensitive nor specific for AIN. White cell casts may be seen on urine microscopy.

A rare hamburger
Then bloody diarrhea
Now little urine

Shiga-Toxin Hemolytic Uremic Syndrome

ST-HUS is a thrombotic microangiopathy limited to the renal vasculature, which presents following an acute bloody diarrheal illness. E. Coli is the most common cause of ST-HUS in industrialized countries with the strain O157:H7 most frequently isolated. Multiple foods have caused outbreaks, though an outbreak in 1993 related to fast-food hamburgers drew enormous public attention. Patients may require dialysis for support but most often will spontaneously recover.

Lifted so much, Bro
For sure, going to be so swole
Dude, check out, red pee

Rhabdomyolysis

Rupture of skeletal muscle membranes with release of myoglobin may either be a global process, as with heat stroke, vigorous exercise, toxins, or infections, including influenza and COVID-19, or more focal, as from prolonged compression of a muscle group during anesthesia or while the patient is intoxicated. Creatine kinase levels are typically markedly elevated. Myoglobulinuria presents as red-pigmented urine but may rapidly progress to severe acute kidney injury from myoglobin tubular toxicity. Hyperkalemia, hyperphosphatemia, and hypocalcemia are common findings. Local muscle injury may produce severe edema, which compresses nerves and blood vessels, resulting in compartment syndrome. (See "Compartment Syndrome")

Feeling off, a cough
Much worse, blood on both tissues
Filling the white bowl
Bloody urine, bloody spit
How were these two fires lit?

Anti-GBM Disease—Goodpasture's

Anti-glomerular basement membrane vasculitis presents with antibodies against the NC1 domain of the alpha 3 chain of type IV collagen. The lungs and kidneys are the exclusive targets with diffuse alveolar hemorrhage, gross hemolysis, and gross hematuria (blood on both tissues, white bowel). This disease can be rapidly morbid or fatal without recognition and prompt treatment. Plasmapheresis to remove the circulating antibody and immunosuppression with glucocorticoids and cyclophosphamide are the most common treatments employed. Patients with Alport's syndrome who receive kidney transplants can develop anti-GBM glomerulonephritis.

Water quality
Center top priority
Dialysis foe
Metal known for neuron woes is
Cleared reverse osmosis

Aluminum Dialysate Contamination

Aluminum is the most abundant metal in the earth's crust. Municipal water supplies can have high aluminum concentrations, which must be removed by reverse osmosis before the water is safe for dialysis use. Chronic aluminum toxicity was common prior to the 1980s when it was discovered that aluminum from water and phosphate binders could cause neurologic and bone disease. Rare acute outbreaks of aluminum contamination still occur, the last reported in Curacao in 2001.

Bacterial grunge
In crystal brushes of sponge
Small cysts turned to stone
Final duct dilatation
Spawns renal rock formation

Medullary Sponge Kidney

Medullary sponge kidney is a congenital malformation of the terminal collecting ducts in the pericalceal region of the renal pyramids. The cystic dilation of distal collecting ducts has a brush-like appearance on CT. The disease is characterized by cyst formation in the medulla (but not the cortex) of the kidneys. There is often nephrocalcinosis and nephrolithiasis. MSK can present with a distal renal tubular acidosis. Typically, renal function is preserved. Patients are treated with potassium citrate to reduce stone formation and treat both acidemia and hypokalemia.

Hyper K trips dance
Ammonia, acid balance
No 3 to make 4
Low aldo means K excess
Block ENAC? Block K egress

Hyperkalemic Renal Tubular Acidosis (Type 4 RTA)

Hyperkalemia impairs ammoniagenesis, ultimately impairing acid clearance as there is no ammonia (NH_3) to be pronated to form ammonium (NH_4). The result is a hyperkalemic metabolic acidosis with a normal serum anion gap and a positive urine anion gap. Etiologies include hyporeninemic hypoaldosteronism and diabetes mellitus. Drugs that can produce a Type 4 RTA include nonsteroid anti-inflammatory drugs (NSAIDs), angiotensin-converting enzyme inhibitors, angiotensin II receptor blockers, spironolactone, heparin, calcineurin inhibitors, and drugs that block the epithelial sodium channel (ENaC) including amiloride, triamterene, and trimethoprim.

Thresholds at cut rate
Spill precious bicarb, phosphate
New sick steady state
All acid, osteo woes
Replete? Out to sea it goes

Fanconi Syndrome with Type 2 Renal Tubular Acidosis

Fanconi syndrome denotes proximal renal tubular dysfunction with reduced thresholds for reabsorption of bicarbonate (type 2 RTA) as well as phosphate, glucose, and amino acids. Fanconi syndrome is often congenital in children but is usually acquired in adults. Light chain nephropathy, Sjogren's syndrome, and heavy metal toxicity can produce Fanconi's syndrome. Vitamin D deficiency, hypophosphatemia, and metabolic acidosis all contribute to the development of osteomalacia. As the resorptive capacity of the proximal tubule is reduced, high dose supplementation is required to overcome losses into the urine.

Beyond winter blues
Sweet, deadly drink to thaw soul
Urine sickly glow
Osmole and anion gaps
Cross lethal paths with time lapse

Ethylene Glycol Poisoning

Ethylene glycol ingestion is usually intentional as part of a suicide attempt and creates an initial osmolar gap. The alcohol dehydrogenase enzyme metabolizes ethylene glycol to oxalic acid, which manifests as an anion gap metabolic acidosis, organ dysfunction, renal failure, and can result in death. As the ethylene glycol is metabolized, the osmolar gap disappears. Fomepizole inhibits alcohol dehydrogenase to prevent conversion to oxalic acid and is typically followed by dialysis for removal. Fluorescein is added to antifreeze, the usual source of ethylene glycol, and results in urine that fluoresces under Wood's lamp after ingestion. Calcium oxalate crystals can be seen on urine microscopy.

Adjust by two days
Brain has nerve-protective ways
When sodium low
Beware water rid too fast
Astrocyte fate may be cast

Osmotic Demyelination Syndrome

Brain cells adjust to hyponatremia by jettisoning solute to limit cellular edema. This process is complete by forty-eight hours, marking the time frame between acute and chronic hyponatremia. Rapid correction (>8mmol/L in twenty-four hours) of hyponatremia that is chronic or of uncertain duration has an increased risk of astrocyte and neuronal injury. Osmotic demyelination syndrome is of highest risk in patients with severe (<105 mmol/L) hyponatremia, concurrent hypokalemia, alcoholism, malnutrition, and cirrhosis.

Thin, weak, sick, headache
Extra strength Q2, I take
Large anion gap

5-Oxoprolinuria/Pyroglutamic Acidosis

5-Oxoprolinuria a.k.a., pyroglutamic acidosis is an under-recognized cause of high anion gap acidosis due to excess acetaminophen ingestion. Patients are typically malnourished, often women, elderly, with glutathione deficiency. Acetaminophen metabolism is shunted to 5-oxoproline, also called pyroglutamic acid. Certain drugs like antiepileptics and flucloxacillin can also precipitate this type of high anion gap acidosis.

Creatinine rise
Do drugs expose or destroy?
Graft pee shows decoy
Dormant virus now awake
Suppressant drugs: time to brake

BK Virus–Associated Nephropathy

The BK virus is a polyoma virus, which is highly endemic, infecting kidney epithelial cells. The infection lies dormant until reactivation in the setting of immunosuppression of a kidney transplant and can cause injurious inflammation to the graft. Decoy cells are BK-virus-infected kidney epithelial cells visible on urine microscopy. Management includes lightening the degree of immunosuppression.

Burnt necrotic plaque
Inner thighs, pannus turned black
Vessels stain like bone
Spent kidneys often, not all
Deadly mark mineral squall

Calciphylaxis

Calciphylaxis is a calcific arteriopathy with exquisitely painful dermal involvement, fat necrosis, and subsequent risk for infection/sepsis. Body areas typically involved include the pannus and the lower extremities at areas of friction, such as between the thighs. The syndrome was initially described in patients with end-stage renal disease (ESRD) but has also been described in non-uremic patients.

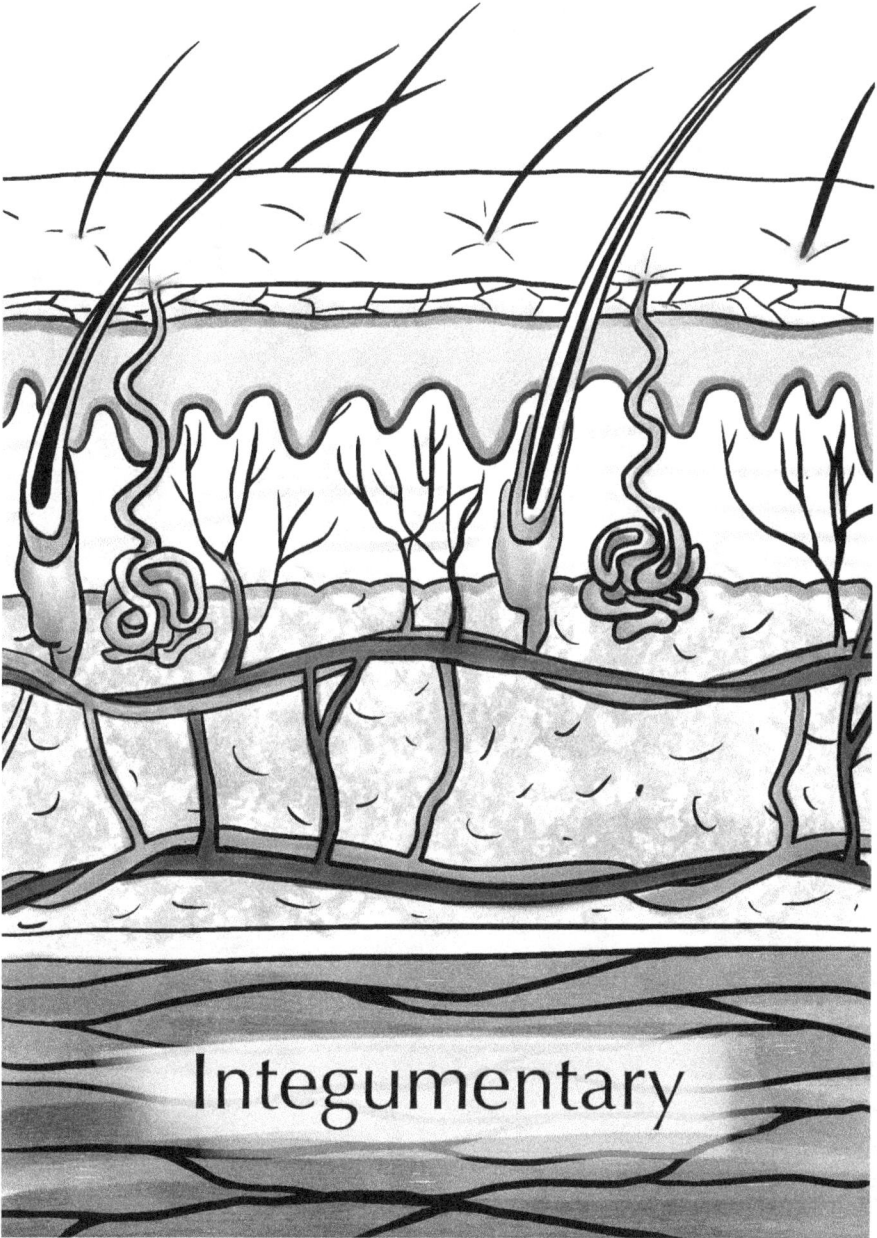
Integumentary

Integumentary
Gaihi

Beyond what you see
These tissues move and cover
All that is inside

"You must play B-ball"
Thumb extends far past your fist
Stretched, lax, and fragile

Marfan Syndrome

Marfan syndrome is an autosomal dominant disorder, usually associated with mutations in *fibrillin* and occasionally with mutations to *TTGFBR1* or *2*. The syndrome has a wide range of clinical manifestations. Tall stature, arachnodactyly (spider fingers), mitral valve prolapse, and importantly, aortic disease are classic features. To slow aortic disease, prophylactic long-acting beta-blockade and/or an angiotensin II receptor blocker (ARB) are recommended. Patients are counseled to avoid high-impact or strenuous exercise.

Turn for the worse, flush
High fevers, a spreading field
Of pinpoint pustules

Acute Generalized Exanthematous Pustulosis

AGEP is primarily a drug eruption that occurs within forty-eight hours of taking an offending medication. It is marked by high fevers, erythematous plaques, and diffuse nonfollicular pustules. It is caused by drug exposure (antibiotics, antimalarials, diltiazem) in 90 percent of cases. The main treatment is to stop the offending medication.

Thick yet bowed with time
Matrix rough, disorganized
Intense on bone scan
High alk phos, bone turnover
Crooked man from crooked dog?

Paget's Disease of Bone

Known historically as osteitis deformans, Paget's disease of bone is a focal disorder of bone metabolism. Affected bone has an accelerated rate of remodeling, which results in disorganized bone overgrowth at single or multiple sites. The affected bone has impaired integrity and is prone to bowing and fractures. Typical sites of involvement include the skull, spine, pelvis, and long bones of the lower extremity. The main symptom is pain and disability due to the bone overgrowth. Bone-specific alkaline phosphatase is usually elevated. The affected bones have intense uptake on bone scintigraphy. Most patients are older than fifty-five years. Animal ownership was initially linked to Paget's but has been since disproved.

Conspicuous flakes
Rain from scalp, now face, trunk, arms
Why all a sudden?

Seborrheic Dermatitis with HIV

Seborrheic dermatitis in immunocompetent people is a chronic, relapsing skin disorder often limited to scaly scalp with typical complaints of dandruff. There may be involvement of the forehead, cheeks, and beard area on men. *Malassezia* fungi may play a role in pathogenesis, particularly in patients with concurrent Parkinson's disease. Patients with HIV and low CD4 counts have increased susceptibility to SD and tend to have more extensive disease, including involvement of the trunk and extremities.

Thick pink-silver scale
Scalp, elbows, gluteal cleft
Nails, a forewarning

Plaque Psoriasis

Psoriasis is a chronic inflammatory skin disease that can manifest in multiple ways. Chronic plaque psoriasis is most common with distinct, erythematous plaques covered by coarse silver scale. Psoriasis may alternatively present as pustules, erythroderma, or the small round plaques known as guttate psoriasis. Plaque psoriasis favors the scalp, extensor surfaces of knees and elbows, and the gluteal cleft. Nail disease is closely associated with psoriatic arthritis.

Legs, dark cool maroon
Thickened skin, woody to touch
Veins have lost their valves

Chronic Venous Stasis Dermatitis

Venous stasis dermatitis arises from venous insufficiency with hyperpigmentation, edema, and scaly thickening of lower leg skin. Patients may present with lipodermatosclerosis with an inverted champagne bottle appearance to their lower leg. Risk factors include female sex, obesity, standing occupation, and a history of deep venous thrombosis. Dysfunction of venous valves is necessary for the pathophysiology. Stasis dermatitis is a mimicker of cellulitis of the legs, though the cracked or scratched skin may become secondarily infected. Deep venous thrombosis and peripheral arterial disease should both be on the differential.

Closed muscle damage
Vessels, nerves wrapped in package
Starved of blood supply

Compartment Syndrome

Compartment syndrome describes acutely raised pressure in a limb muscle compartment, which is constrained by fascial membranes. The lower leg anterior compartment is most often affected and may be due to tibial fracture, blunt injury, or vascular trauma. The pressure in the compartment compresses and halts blood flow, causing an ischemic injury to the muscles and nerves. The five *P*s often described, e.g., pallor, paresthesia, loss of pulsation, pain with passive motion, and pain out of proportion are late signs of compartment syndrome. The intervention required for compartment syndrome is emergent fasciotomy to lower pressures and limit injury.

Lysine proline off
Unwise sailor will just scoff
Fate filled with bruises
God save ye teeth in yer prime
Orange squeeze, lemon splash, juiced lime

Scurvy

Vitamin C is a necessary cofactor for hydroxylation of lysine and proline, both important components of collagen. Unlike some animals, humans are unable to synthesize vitamin C. Deficiency of this vitamin leads to significant gum disease with potential for tooth loss, hyperkeratosis of skin, and capillary fragility. In 1747, surgeon James Lind on the HMS *Salisbury* completed one of the first clinical trials, giving half his affected sailors citrus juice and fruits and the other half vinegar, cider, and horseradish. The sailors receiving citrus quickly recovered. British ships were subsequently required to carry citrus fruits, gaining British sailors the nickname limeys.

Hurry time to go!
Hasty arm grab, prone elbow
Yet more parent guilt

Nursemaid's Elbow

Radial head subluxation, typically in a child under the age of five, can occur after the child's arm is grabbed or swung. The child with nursemaid's elbow refuses to use the arm and holds the arm close to the body, slightly prone and extended. The radial head can usually be reduced quickly and without the need for anesthesia.

Dense neuropathy
Ankle foot no sense of space
Bones crush in awkward place

Charcot Neuropathic Arthropathy (Charcot Joint)

Charcot neuropathy arthropathy is joint deformity/destruction, typically of the foot and ankle, due to a large peripheral fiber neuropathy such as diabetes mellitus, vitamin B12 deficiency, syphilis, copper deficiency, or dorsal column dysfunction. The dense neuropathy leads to repeated trauma, presenting either as an acute, hot joint or more insidious accumulation of deformity. The rocker-bottom foot is a classic appearance of an advanced Charcot joint.

Comes, goes suddenly
Pink, peel, shape, scale, Christmas tree
Hark to the herald

Pityriasis Rosea

Pityriasis rosea is a cutaneous eruption of unclear etiology that starts with a mother or herald patch. The patch typically has a raised border and is pruritic with fine scale. The rash progresses along the Langer (cleavage) lines of the trunk and limbs in a fir tree pattern. Patients may develop malaise, fatigue, nausea, joint pain, fever, and sore throat before or during the rash. The rash is self-limited with a mean duration of forty-five days.

More than a boxer's
Nose has bled, no punch needed
Purple dots the lips

Hereditary Hemorrhagic Telangiectasia (Osler Weber Rendu)

Hereditary hemorrhagic telangiectasia is an autosomal dominant vascular disorder characterized by recurrent epistaxis, gastrointestinal bleeding, systemic arteriovenous malformations, and diffuse mucocutaneous telangiectasias (lips, tongue, buccal mucosa, fingers). Bleeding and telangiectasias typically begin in young adulthood and increase with age.

Gynecology
& Genitourinary

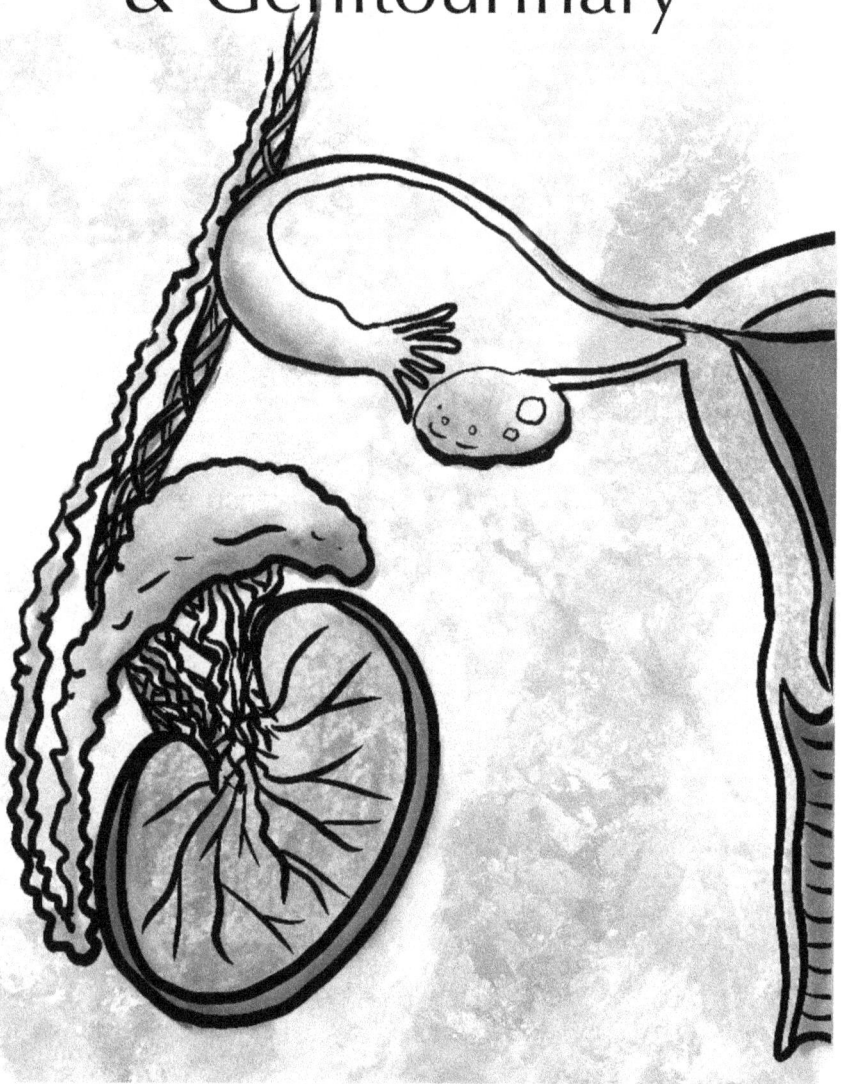

Genitourinary/Gynecology
Hinyoseishokuki/Fujin-ka

Kept for self, lovers
Focused relief, shame, pleasure
Creation of life

Love to love you, but
Fish? Our chemistry smells off
Wish we had a clue

Bacterial Vaginosis

Bacterial vaginosis is a common cause of vaginal discharge in premenopausal women. It is associated with sexual activity—both for heterosexual women and women who have sex with women (WSW). The symptoms are due to a shift in the vaginal flora from lactobacillus to a variety of flora including Gardnerella. Symptoms include a fish odor but no pain or dyspareunia. The diagnosis is made by finding vaginal secretions with increased pH, whiff test with KOH, and clue cells (epithelial cells coated with Gardnerella organisms) on microscopy.

Calcium, once friend
Now complex, wedged, a sharp cork
The squeeze is savage

Calcium Ureterolithiasis

Calcium urinary stones are the most common type of kidney stones with calcium oxalate more frequent than calcium phosphate. The stone forms in the kidney on a papillary structure called Randall's plaque. It grows and eventually breaks free to traverse the ureteral system. The colicky pain of a stone too big to pass easily through the ureter (sharp cork) is, by report, excruciating and produces colicky flank pain with the ureter's peristalsis.

Lust's ironic end
Such exquisite tenderness
Has few equal peers
On bimanual exam
Reaching for chandeliers

Pelvic Inflammatory Disease

PID is an infection of the upper tract of gynecologic organs, mostly with sexually transmitted infections such as gonorrhea and chlamydia. Patients can have significant cervical motion tenderness on exam (the chandelier sign) and may have metastatic infection, which involves the hepatic capsule (Fitz-Hugh-Curtis syndrome). PID involves a risk of tuboovarian abscess with sepsis. Tubes scarred by PID may result in infertility.

Escape womb artist
Setting up shop where you land
Cycles of distress

Endometriosis

Endometriosis is the result of ectopic endometrial cells implanting, growing, and creating an inflammatory response. Lesions are typically in the pelvis—on the uterus, ovaries, bladder, rectum—but can occur throughout the abdominal and pleural cavities. The most common pathogenic theory (Sampson's theory) is that endometrial cells move retrograde from the uterus through the fallopian tubes to the peritoneal cavity during menstruation. Symptoms include dysmenorrhea, dyspareunia, chronic pain, and infertility. Bowel involvement can lead to symptoms of diarrhea and constipation. The growth of the implants is driven by estrogen and the menstrual cycle.

Tiny coffin lids
Craggy peaks, bugs hide amid
Growth is so basic

Struvite Nephrolithiasis

Struvite, or magnesium ammonium phosphate stones, are strongly associated with urease-producing bacteria. These bacteria infect both urine and stones and produce a high pH (basic) environment, which promotes stone growth. These stones often take the shape of the urinary system, forming craggy staghorn calculi. Urine crystals look like coffin lids under urine microscopy.

Lugging this belly
A chore, sore back, puffy hands
Makes my BP rise

Preeclampsia

Preeclampsia is a peripartum vasculopathy characterized by the development of new-onset hypertension and proteinuria after twenty weeks of gestation. Lower extremity edema is common in pregnancy, but hand and face edema suggest preeclampsia. Headaches and visual symptoms are alarming symptoms and may herald onset of eclampsia and seizures. Obesity (>30 BMI), nulliparity, maternal age older than thirty-five years, multifetal gestations, and assisted reproductive technologies are all associated with increased risk of preeclampsia. IV magnesium appears to lower risk of progression to eclampsia, which manifests as seizures. Delivery is the definitive treatment.

Once a straight shooter
Too much love, now too much curve
Mojo without means

Peyronie's Disease

Peyronie's is a common urological complaint of men, with more than one in ten reporting symptoms. Minor trauma to the penis can lead to progressive scarring, curvature, and dysfunction. This curve can result in significant loss of sexual satisfaction for the patient and his partner. The disease is named for Francois Gigot de la Peyronie, the physician to French king Louis XV.

Whorled growths of unclear need
Deform womb bulk, increase bleed
Tight fetal quarters

Uterine Leiomyoma or Fibroids

Uterine leiomyomas or fibroids are benign tumors of smooth muscles and fibroblasts that have a whorled appearance on cut surface. The tumors are estrogen-dependent. The main symptoms are bulk, pressure and heavy menstrual bleeding. Fibroids may interfere with fertility and increase the risk of miscarriage.

Erratic cycle
Acne, can that be a beard?
Hard to lose this weight

Polycystic Ovarian Syndrome

PCOS is a disease of adolescent girls and women that features clinical signs of androgen excess and insulin resistance. Polycystic ovaries alone are insufficient to make the diagnosis. Symptoms may include hirsutism, acne vulgaris, menstrual irregularities, acanthosis nigricans, and obesity. Hirsutism is defined as excess sexual hair growth in a male pattern. Many patients with PCOS will have metabolic syndrome. Patients should undergo a broad evaluation for other causes of hyperadrogenism.

Slow strangulation
Engulfing the ureters
Dull ache of hydro

Retroperitoneal Fibrosis

Retroperitoneal fibrosis is rare periaortic inflammation, fibrosis, and strangulation of the retroperitoneal structures. RPF is on the differential for postrenal kidney failure. Medial displacement of the ureters can be seen on imaging along with ill-defined masses of fibrous and desmoplastic tissue. Ureteral patency is a priority. RPF is primarily thought to be idiopathic, though it may be related to IgG4, malignancy, or certain drugs (including ergots).

Chronic case of runs
Exquisite pain, stuck stone stuns
KUB stone-free

Uric Acid Nephrolithiasis

Uric acid stones are radiolucent and so not seen on plain films such as a KUB. They are often seen in patients with chronic diarrhea who produce low volume, low pH urine. They are also seen in high uric acid states, including gout and patients with rapid cell turnover, such as leukemia, myeloproliferative neoplasia, psoriasis. Treatment includes addressing the underlying predisposing disorder, alkalinizing the urine, and increasing fluid intake.

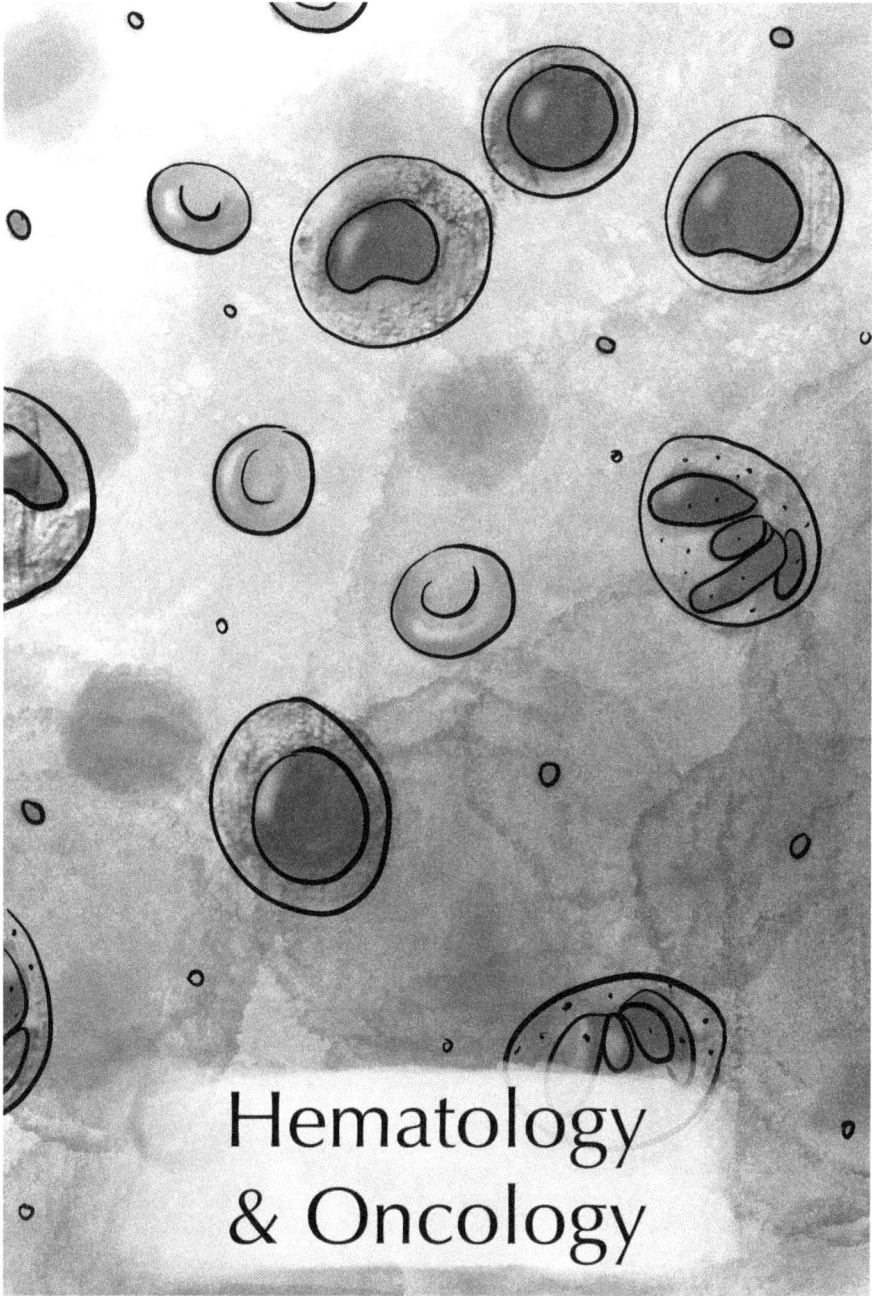

Hematology
& Oncology

Hematology/Oncology
Ketsueki-gaku/Shuyo-gaku

Red, blue, white, flowing
Or cells gone rogue; both involve
One's immunity

Acute swollen leg
Firm balloon at liver's edge
Sclera tinged yellow

Pancreatic Cancer with Eponymous Signs

The clinical presentation is one of a pancreatic head mass adenocarcinoma with (1) painless jaundice; (2) Courvoisier's sign of an enlarged, palpable gallbladder in that setting; and (3) Trousseau's sign of malignant hypercoagulability with the presence of deep vein thrombosis. Cure of pancreatic adenocarcinoma depends on whether the tumor can be surgically resected, e.g., through a Whipple surgery, either at the time of diagnosis or following neoadjuvant therapy.

Why would red mass grow?
Smoking? No. Altitude? No.
Tumor EPO? No.
Such an itch in warm water
Red hands, feet feel pain, hotter

Polycythemia Vera

Polycythemia vera is a myeloproliferative neoplasm resulting in increased red cell mass. The differential diagnosis includes other causes of polycythemia, including smoking, reduced oxygen tension, and exogenous or endogenous (e.g., renal cell carcinoma) erythropoietin. The marked elevation in red cell mass can cause headache, visual symptoms, and stroke. Aquagenic pruritus and erythromelalgia (red, painful hands and feet) are classic signs of PV.

Intrinsic pathway malign
Bloody circumcision sign
Disease of princes
Victoria regal source
End of Russian czarist course

Hemophilia B

Hemophilia B (also known as Christmas disease) is X-linked factor IX deficiency, a crucial part of the intrinsic pathway. Like patients with hemophilia A (factor VIII deficiency), patients present with epistaxis, hemarthrosis, and excessive bleeding, including hemorrhage with circumcision. Queen Victoria was a carrier and passed the gene onto three of her nine children. Her great-grandson Alexei, the only son of Czar Nicholas II of Russia, was affected by the disease. He died by firing squad with the rest of his family. The mutated gene for factor IX was sequenced from his remains.

Fast-growing tumor
Mass mitosis, ill humor
Outstrips blood supply
Leaks of phosphate, urate
Garbage in the kidneys' grates

Tumor Lysis Syndrome

Tumor lysis syndrome is an oncologic emergency due to cell lysis, either spontaneously with fast-growing malignancies such as acute lymphoblastic leukemia, Burkitt's lymphoma, or diffuse large B cell lymphoma, or after the initiation of chemotherapy. Cell lysis results in a flood of intracellular contents being spilled into the circulation with resultant hyperkalemia, hyperphosphatemia (and subsequent hypocalcemia), and hyperuricemia. Patients may develop arrhythmias and rapid onset oliguric or anuric acute kidney injury.

M lambda light chain
Darkened, swollen skin, weak, pain
Hormone function off
VEGF above-normal zone
Osteosclerotic bone

POEMS syndrome

POEMS is an acronym for polyneuropathy, organomegaly, endocrinopathy, monoclonal protein, skin changes. The syndrome is now characterized by major criteria, including polyneuropathy and monoclonal (almost always lambda) plasma cell dyscrasia. Other major criteria include Castleman disease, elevated vascular endothelial growth factor (VEGF), and sclerotic bone lesions. There are broad minor criteria including skin hyperpigmentation, hypertrichosis, edema, and endocrine dysfunction. There is no standard treatment for POEMS though treatment of advanced disease is like that of multiple myeloma.

Crowding out all good
Blasts blast into marrowhood
Hot-pink rod gang sign

Acute Myeloid Leukemia

Acute myeloid leukemia (AML) is the most common acute leukemia in adults with the median age of diagnosis approximately sixty-five years. A classic presentation is pancytopenia in the elderly patient with symptoms of fatigue and weakness. Peripheral blood shows circulating blasts and the bone marrow biopsy shows a hypercellular marrow that is crowded by leukemic cells. Blasts show Auer rods, which mark their myeloid origin.

Small change chemistry
Cruel loss pliability
Wide-range infarctions
Hypoxia, searing pain
Brief control, begin again

Sickle Cell Anemia

A single point mutation in the beta chain of hemoglobin results in the mutant hemoglobin S (HbS), which, when homozygous, is prone to polymerization and sickling in the setting of hypoxemia and acidosis. Red cells are deformed into a poorly compliant sickle shape, which can lodge in small blood vessels and cause vasoocclusive crises. Patients have lifelong episodes of pain from both acute and chronic infarctions. They are at risk for infections due to functional asplenia and are at increased risk of stroke and pregnancy complications. The clinical picture is modified when one HbS gene is heterozygous with other hemoglobin mutants such as thalassemia.

Packed strands give a sheen
Birefringent, apple green
To stiff, stuffed organs

AL Amyloidosis

AL amyloidosis is due to a clonal disease of plasma cells, which produce light chains capable of tissue deposition and disruption. Widespread organ damage ranges from liver and heart injury to nephrotic syndrome and Fanconi's syndrome. Patients may have hyperglossia or vascular fragility with easy bruising. Serum protein electrophoresis and serum free light chains may show a clonal population. Tissue diagnosis is achieved through fat pad biopsy or biopsy of involved organ showing apple-green birefringence under Congo red stain.

Fevers like clockwork
Spike each day, bed drenched each night
"Swollen glands," mono?

Hodgkin's Lymphoma

Fever, night sweats, lymphadenopathy are all hallmarks of Hodgkin's lymphoma—though rheumatologic and infectious etiologies would be on the differential. The haiku suggests a fever pattern consistent with Pel Ebstein fever—one associated with Hodgkin's lymphoma—of daily fevers that rise and fall over the course of weeks. The Reed Sternberg (owl eye) cells are distinctive giant cells found on lymph node biopsy in patients with Hodgkin's.

All vicinity
Bound with tight affinity
Space heater on fritz
Whole house red, barely alive
Force free heme with long deep dive

Carbon Monoxide Poisoning

Carbon monoxide is colorless, odorless gas associated with poorly functioning or ventilated heaters, furnaces, and engines. CO has significantly higher affinity than O_2 for the heme molecule and is able to bind tightly, leading to cellular hypoxia. CO-bound heme is red, and patients will appear flushed and have normal O_2 saturation readings. The treatment is 100 percent oxygen delivered either a normal pressure or through a hyperbaric chamber (deep dive) to displace CO from heme. Treatment with hyperbaric 100 percent oxygen may have better long-term neurologic outcomes.

Red pee each morning
Low haptoglobin warning
Complement run wild
Sudden painful liver clot
Cell surface defense is shot

Paroxysmal Nocturnal Hemoglobinuria

PNH is due to an acquired deficiency in cell surface protective proteins CD55/CD59 due to mutations in the *PIGA* gene, essential for synthesis of their anchor proteins. Red cells are left undefended against the membrane attack complex of complement and are lysed, typically at times of lower oxygen tension or pH, hence the title nocturnal. Hemoglobin binds to haptoglobin, reducing its level, and can spill into the urine as red hemoglobinuria. Patients are also prone to hypercoagulability and thrombosis of major veins, including the hepatic vein (causing Budd Chiari syndrome), mesenteric veins, central venous sinus, and other deep veins. PNH can be a precursor to aplastic anemia, myelodysplastic syndrome, and leukemias.

White clots starve, smother
Stop heparin, start other
Assay PF4

Heparin-Induced Thrombocytopenia (HIT)

HIT results from an immunologic reaction to the complex of heparin and platelet factor 4. The clinical presentation ranges from low platelet counts to widespread venous and arterial thrombosis with platelet-rich white clots. Diagnosis requires clinical evaluation with the 4T score and a biologic assay such as the heparin-PF4/serotonin release assay. HIT is a pro-thrombotic state that requires discontinuation of all heparin products and the start of alternative systemic anticoagulation.

Tried Atkins diet
Cramping intense belly pain
So weak, dark urine
Dextrose provides temp relief
Hemin resolves pain motif

Porphyria

Complex series of diseases related to abnormal hemoglobin formation. Acute intermittent porphyria is a rare autosomal dominant enzyme deficiency that interferes with hemoglobin synthesis. It is the most common acute porphyria. Women are affected more often than men. AIP presents with abdominal pain and nausea/vomiting but also neurologic symptoms of peripheral neuropathy, psychiatric symptoms, and seizures. Dark or red urine may be observed. Low carbohydrate diets (like the Atkins diet) or starvation are triggers. Dextrose infusion can be a temporizing treatment to stem symptoms, but IV hemin is the definitive therapy required to resolve an attack.

Cancer, infection
Traumatic obstetric end
What sparked this whirlwind
Platelets, fibrin splintered heap
Oust source before in too deep

Disseminated Intravascular Coagulation (DIC)

DIC is due to the diffuse activation of platelets and fibrin, through exposure to tissue factor, resulting in a cascade of thrombosis and bleeding. The trigger is usually acute, such as an infection or an obstetric catastrophe, though cancer can produce a more subacute/chronic picture of DIC. There is evidence of microangiopathic hemolytic anemia and a thrombotic microangiopathy. Elevation of PT and aPTT differentiates DIC from other thrombotic microangiopathies such as thrombotic thrombocytopenia (TTP) and hemolytic uremic syndrome (HUS). Treatment involves identifying and removing the inciting factor and additional supportive management, including transfusions if needed.

Purple ears and nose
Ulcers at sites of Raynaud
Cool hemolysis
Ere more tissue be fodder
Send sample in warm water

Cold Agglutinin Disease

Cold agglutinin disease is an autoimmune hemolytic anemia with antibodies active at cold temperatures. Symptoms include Coombs positive extravascular hemolysis, acrocyanosis, livedo, Raynaud's phenomenon, and necrosis. Pain with ingestion of cold food is a common symptom. The disease is associated with mycoplasma and EBV infections and with lymphoid malignancies.

One eyelid drooping
A cough that will not quit, blood?
Dry face, small pupil

Horner Syndrome

The syndrome is a combination of ptosis (drooping lid), meiosis (small pupil), and anhidrosis (sweat-free skin) seen in injury or invasion of the ipsilateral sympathetic nervous system stellate ganglion. The findings represent a loss of sympathetic activity. There are multiple reported etiologies though invasion of the ganglion by an apical lung cancer (a Pancoast tumor) is a classic presentation.

Liquid shrinks the lungs
They extract, yet it comes back
Shards dot the pleura
Remote navy service risks
Hard work spent changing brake disks

Malignant Mesothelioma

Mesothelioma is a malignancy arising from either the thoracic pleura or the abdominal peritoneum. There is a strong association with asbestos exposure as well as with smoking. Asbestos exposure is primarily occupation related such as shipbuilding and work with friction materials, such as brake pads and gaskets. The cancer may present with pleuritic chest pain but often presents as a recurrent and progressive exudative pleural effusion. Cytology may be inconclusive from thoracentesis and pleural biopsy may be necessary for diagnosis. Benign asbestos-related pleural effusion (BAPE) is on the differential but without evidence or development of malignancy.

A hard left neck lump
Pale, thin, an ill-defined ache
Barely touch my plate

Virchow's Node (Stomach Cancer)

Virchow's node, or the left supraclavicular node, marks the site where the thoracic duct empties into the left subclavian vein. Malignant involvement of this lymph node heralds an intra-abdominal malignancy. The poem features early satiety, anemia, and weight loss, suggesting a stomach cancer as the source of the Virchow's node.

Pneumonia, cough
Red counts low, kidneys are off
Such pain in my bones

Multiple Myeloma

Multiple myeloma is a malignancy of plasma cells that produce a monoclonal immunoglobulin. The malignant cells proliferate in bone and can cause extensive bony damage through osteolytic lesions and pathologic fractures. Other key features are hypercalcemia, renal injury, and anemia—rounding out the CRAB mnemonic. Anemia is the most common sign followed by bone pain. Patients are at increased risk for infections due to suppression of normal immunoglobulin production.

Sudden bloom again
Flat crops of pinpoint red marks
Very few platelets

Immune Thrombocytopenia

Adult ITP is often recurrent with the emergence, disappearance, and reemergence of an IgG antibody against platelets. The low platelet count tilts the body's normal homeostatic balance toward bleeding. Small nonblanching petechiae appear on the lower extremities more than on the upper extremities. The risk of intracranial bleeding goes up with falling counts though does not precipitously rise until counts <10K. Steroids and intravenous immunoglobulin (IVIG) are common first line agents for treatment.

Destroyed intrinsic
Tongue sore, pale conjunctiva
Lemon-yellow hue

Pernicious Anemia (Vitamin B12 Deficiency [Hematology/Oncology])

Pernicious anemia is an autoimmune cause of vitamin B12 deficiency due to autoantibodies to intrinsic factor, gastric parietal cells, or both. Patients typically present with macrocytic anemia, lemon-yellow skin from anemia and jaundice, and variable neurologic symptoms. Vitamin B12 can cause glossitis with a red, smooth, painful tongue. Intrinsic factor antibodies identify the disease as autoimmune. Treatment includes parenteral B12 repletion. (See "Vitamin B12 Deficiency (Neurology/Psychiatry)")

Clonal giant *M*
Congregates and chokes off flow
Each centipoise slows

Waldenstrom's Macroglobulinemia

Waldenstrom's macroglobulinemia is a low-grade B-cell lymphoproliferative disorder heralded by production of monoclonal IgM. The proteins can deposit in tissues as amyloid (liver, nerve) but also can cause hyperviscosity syndrome. Hyperviscosity, measured in centipoise, manifests as headaches and visual changes.

Neurology
& Psychiatry

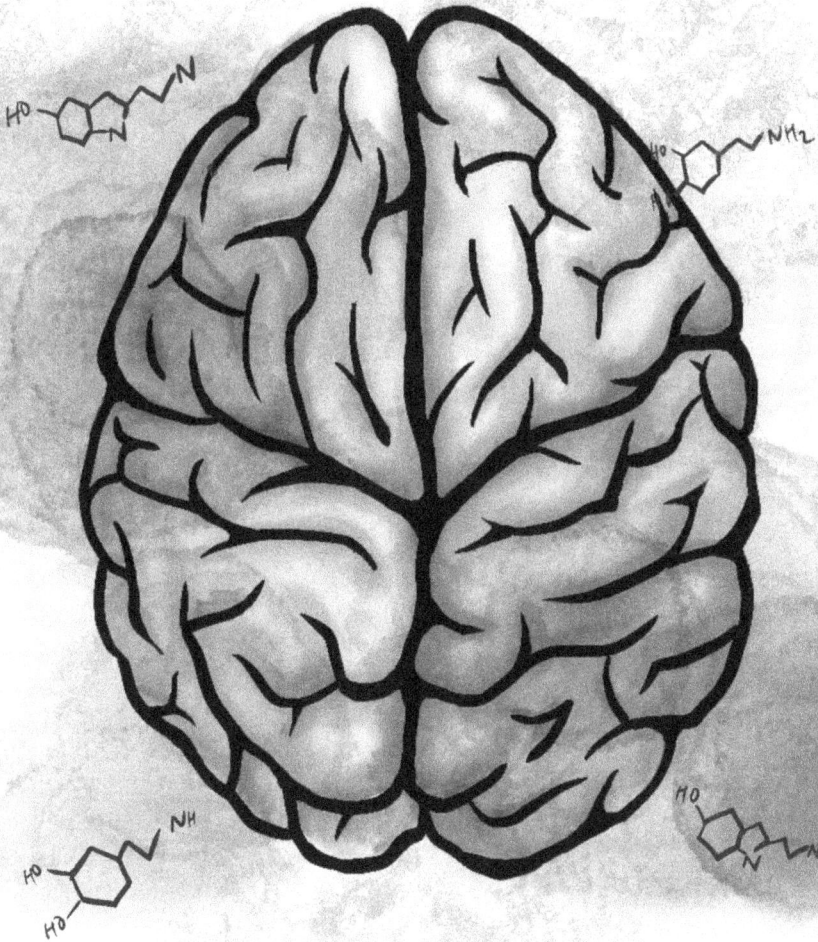

Neurology/Psychiatry
Shinkei seishin igaku

You are all you know
Observations black and white
The soul adds color

My eye an icepick
Each 3 a.m., seconds tick
The tears are my tell

Cluster Headache

Cluster headaches are considered one of the most painful primary headaches syndromes, e.g., suicide headaches. They are more common in men, typically unilateral and associated with lacrimation. Patients' headaches will cluster with a stereotypical pattern of headaches at the same time of day, often waking from sleep, with crescendo to several headaches a day and then be gone for months or years at a time. In this way, the headaches both cluster at a particular time and in discrete episodes lasting days to weeks at a time. Typical migraine medications have limited efficacy in aborting and treating these headaches. The best abortive therapy is oxygen. Diagnosis is often delayed by years.

Diarrhea gone
But now I trip, I stumble
So tough to swallow
Weakness ascends from below
Check the force of the bellows

Guillain-Barre Syndrome

GBS is an immune-mediated polyneuropathy, commonly presenting as an acute, acquired weakness, often following a preceding infection. The infection may be a diarrheal illness (classically with the bacteria *Campylobacter*) though GBS has been described after respiratory infections and influenza-like illnesses, including influenza A and B, CMV, and COVID-19. Typical clinical features include progressive, symmetric muscle weakness, and absent or depressed deep tendon reflexes. Weakness usually begins in the legs and ascends. Paresthesia of the hands and feet are common, as is back pain and autonomic dysfunction. Respiratory muscle weakness may result in a need for ventilatory support.

Room thrown into spin
Poor PO save liquor in
Ophthalmoplegia
Think twice before pulse dextrose
Ere give thiamine high dose

Wernicke's Encephalopathy

Severe thiamine (vitamin B1) deficiency causes the classic triad of confusion, ataxia, and ophthalmoplegia. The syndrome is often described with severe alcoholism, but increasingly as a complication of weight loss surgery, as well as malnutrition and anorexia nervosa. When glucose is given prior to repletion of thiamine, the symptoms of deficiency are exacerbated as stores are further depleted. Treatment requires IV administration of high dose thiamine.

Fatigue drapes heavy
My wide mediastinum
So hard to look up

Myasthenia Gravis

Myasthenia gravis is an autoimmune neurological disease presenting with fatigue, ocular weakness, and often more generalized weakness (including facial, bulbar, respiratory). Weakness is often worsened by activity. A thymoma (causing a wide mediastinum) is present in 10–15 percent of patients. Treatment includes thymectomy (if thymoma is present) and long-term immunosuppressant medications. The first reported case was likely Native American chief Opechancanough, who died in 1664 with historic accounts describing classic findings of fatigue and eyelids that needed to be lifted by attendants.

Too much dentist fun
Feet, hands clumsy, thick, and numb
Painful party end

Vitamin B12 Deficiency (Neurology/Psychiatry)

Nitrous oxide, or laughing gas, is typically delivered as anesthesia for medical or dental procedures but may be used recreationally through inhalation of N_2O canisters called whippets. Nitrous oxide inactivates vitamin B12 and impairs its ability to act as cofactor for methionine synthase. B12 levels may appear normal to low normal, and diagnosis requires testing of homocysteine and methylmalonic acid to reveal the deficiency. As with B12 deficiency of any kind, symptoms may range from anemia to neurologic and psychiatric symptoms. (See "Pernicious Anemia (Vitamin B12 Deficiency [Hematology/Oncology])")

Fading nigra takes
Fluidity, expression
A tremor persists
Shuffling but not like a dance
Letters shrink, as does my stance

Idiopathic Parkinson's Disease

Parkinson's disease (PD) is a degenerative neurologic disease marked by a resting pill-rolling tremor, bradykinesia, akinesia, postural instability, rigidity, and a shuffling gait. The substantia nigra and other dopaminergic structures of the brain show degeneration and loss of dark pigmentation. Handwriting and repeated movements (e.g., finger-tapping) becoming smaller and reduced facial expression are common features of the disease. Orthostatic hypotension can be a prominent feature of PD and makes treatment with carbidopa/levodopa more difficult as the medication can exacerbate these symptoms.

Mind all a twitter
Erratic burst of wit, their
Brain needs a sitter
Interrupting, no filter
Lithium can quell the spell

Hypomania

Hypomania is a feature of bipolar disorder 2 and presents as a distinct period of abnormally elevated or irritable mood with increased activity or energy and decreased need for sleep. The hypomanic patient presents as more talkative or pressured in speech, with frequent interrupting. They have racing ideas, distractibility, and typically an increase in goal-directed activity (e.g., toward work or school, writing, composing, etc.). Hypomania is less severe than full-blown mania, and there is no psychosis (i.e., abnormal thinking, delusions or hallucinations). Substance abuse is on the differential as is the effect of anti-depressant medications. Lithium salts are often used for mood stabilization in the treatment of bipolar disorder.

Right? Left? Double view
Each nod sends electric shock
Summer makes it worse

Multiple Sclerosis

Seen more often in young women than men, multiple sclerosis is a chronic diffuse demyelinating disease of the central nervous system, which can have either a remitting and relapsing or progressive course. Blurry vision, double vision and eye movement abnormalities, including intranuclear ophthalmoplegia with paralysis of abducting gaze and subsequent horizontal nystagmus are common symptoms and signs of MS. L'Hermitte's sign, an electric shock felt in the body with nod of the head, is classic but not specific for multiple sclerosis. Uhthoff's phenomenon describes the worsening of symptoms when the patient is overheated, such as after exiting a warm shower or in warm summer months.

So I'm going to end
Can't accept performing sad
World so dark, unkind

Unipolar Major Depression

Major depression is a common psychiatric disorder with complex and myriad presentations and is a leading cause of disability around the world. The disorder is typically characterized by persistent depressed or dysphoric mood. The haiku contains the mnemonic SIG E CAPS—sleep changes, loss of interest, guilt, lack of energy, loss of cognition or concentration, changes in appetite, psychomotor changes, and suicidal preoccupation—that is often used to evaluate for and characterize the mood disorder. No one patient, though, must have all the referenced elements for the diagnosis to be made. There may be comorbidity with anxiety disorder, substance use disorder, obsessive compulsive disorder, and post-traumatic stress disorder.

Brittle, closed in
As cast by Madame Tussaud
Benzos thaw the freeze

Catatonia

Catatonia is often a complication of a severe underlying mood or psychotic disorder. Signs include mutism, rigidity, negativism, echopraxia, echolalia and waxy (Madame Tussaud) flexibility. Drug-induced Parkinsonism should be considered in the differential diagnosis, especially in patients with mood or psychotic disorders taking antipsychotics. The malignant variant of catatonia can look like neuroleptic malignant syndrome. Rarely, catatonia may present with a hyperactive variant. Catatonia typically responds well to benzodiazepines and electroconvulsive therapy.

Work in garden shed
Broken ventilation head
Almost left for dead
Crying, brisk salivation
Belladonna salvation

Cholinesterase Inhibitor Poisoning

Cholinesterase inhibitors (e.g., organophosphate, carbamate) are used as insecticides and may be found in household gardening products. Poisoning presents with overactivation of the parasympathetic nervous system and symptoms including salivation, diarrhea, vomiting, lacrimation, small pupils, tremors, seizures and confusion. Atropine (derived from the belladonna plant) and pralidoxime are antidotes. Most cases of poisoning occur in those working in agriculture and the drugs have also been used in suicide attempts. Treatment may require repeated doses of the antidote.

Hot, restless, stiff, rude
Wrong turn, drugs meant to lift mood
"Happy" signal storm

Serotonin Syndrome

Serotonin syndrome has a variable presentation ranging from relatively benign to deadly and is diagnosed in patients with a history of exposure to one or more serotonergic drugs. Patients show altered mental status, restlessness, hyperthermia, agitation, hyperreflexia, and clonus. The onset is rapid as compared with neuroleptic malignant syndrome. The Hunter criteria may aid diagnosis. Management consists of immediate discontinuation of serotonergic agents, hydration, and supportive care. Patients may require sedation with benzodiazepines.

Disrupt the whole school
Play with fire, break every rule
Kick your sister's cat
Rob a store and shoot the clerk
The jail toughs call you a jerk

Antisocial Personality Disorder

Antisocial personality disorder is marked by a disregard for norms and the rights of others. Those affected often show exploitive and criminal behavior marked by a lack of remorse. Unemployment and incarceration are frequent outcomes, as is an inability to form stable relationships. Antisocial personal disorder cannot be diagnosed in childhood with similar behavior classified as conduct disorder in children.

Encasing the nerve
Muffling sound along each curve
Boring into bone

Acoustic Neuroma

Acoustic neuroma or vestibular schwannoma is a benign tumor of Schwann cells and accounts for one in twelve intracranial tumors in adults. The usual location is with cranial nerve VIII at the cerebellopontine angle. Patients typically present with unilateral hearing loss but may also have imbalance and mass effect on adjacent structures. The leading differential diagnosis is a meningioma.

Heart pounding in ears
Breaths so ragged, unknown threat
Hands curl into fists
With every gulp, pH raised
Can't feel face, I must look crazed

Panic Attack with Hyperventilation

A panic attack is a discrete episode of intense fear typically lasting for minutes which typically presents as sudden onset of anxiety, a feeling of dread or doom, an urge to escape, chest tightness or pain. The attack may happen alone or as part of underling psychiatric or medical disorder. Disordered breathing with hyperventilation is a common manifestation of the attack. Hyperventilation leads to respiratory alkalosis with subsequent freeing up of binding sites on negatively charged serum albumin. Free calcium ions bind to these sites, creating transient hypocalcemia. Extracellular potassium also exchanges for intracellular hydrogen ions, resulting in transient hypokalemia. Sequelae and symptoms of these electrolyte abnormalities can range from perioral paresthesia, carpopedal spasm, trismus to arrhythmias.

Rapid loss of self
Warped proteins poison, punch holes
Startled by the pace

Creutzfeldt-Jakob Disease

CJD is a rapidly progressive fatal degenerative brain disorder named after German neurologists Hans Gerhard Creutzfeldt and Alfons Maria Jakob. CJD is a prion disease in which misfolded proteins cause normal proteins to become misfolded through a chain reaction. Typical symptoms include progressive memory loss, personality changes, behavioral and executive function issues, and hallucinations. Startle myoclonus is a clinical feature of most patients. EEG typically shows triphasic discharges and a characteristic MRI finding is cortical diffusion restriction named the cortical-ribbon sign. There is no specific treatment, and most patients die within one year of symptom onset.

Soon I'll be found out
Peers so smart and ambitious
I'm here by mistake

Imposter Phenomenon

Imposter phenomenon is a pattern of negative, persistent and pervasive thinking in which the individual doubts their skill, intelligence, and self-worthiness, and thereby operates under a fear of being exposed as an imposter or a fraud. Recent research has begun to characterize imposter phenomenon in various population groups, including medical students, women, and people who represent a racial, ethnic or sexual minority. Imposter phenomenon may be higher among individuals who are high-achieving and does not necessarily correlate with objective competence. Various interventions have been proposed, including mentorship, focusing on self-worth and resilience, and individual and group psychotherapy.

Whether the type who
Would mull over a haiku
Or just for teaching
Hope much was learned, good time won
Thanks for being part of fun

ACKNOWLEDGMENTS

Thank you to the incredibly thoughtful and generous Massachusetts General Hospital resident physicians who helped to refine the poems and assure the explanations were accurate: Dr. Hayden Andrews, Dr. Jose Castellanos, Dr. Vladislav Fomin, Dr. Galina Gheihman, Dr. Stefanie Gerstberger, Dr. Shauna Newton, Dr. Krishna Pandya, Dr. Daria Schatoff, and Dr. Zandra Walton.

Thank you to Sadaharu Honda for the Japanese translation.

Thank you lastly to my remarkable children, who may never want to read a haiku again. You have been incredibly tolerant. I love you with all my heart.

INDEX

CPSIA information can be obtained
at www.ICGtesting.com
Printed in the USA
LVHW040227300622
722004LV00002BA/2

9 781669 810018